The Power of Positive Aging

To Melinda + Phil—
Long ago friends—
Best love,
Donna!

The Power of Positive Aging

Seeing Life as a Glorious Voyage

Donna Devall

Library of Congress Control Number:		2010901135
ISBN:	Hardcover	978-1-4500-3436-4
	Softcover	978-1-4500-3435-7
	Ebook	978-1-4500-3437-1

This book was printed in the United States of America.

To order additional copies of this book, contact:
Xlibris Corporation
1-888-795-4274
www.Xlibris.com
Orders@Xlibris.com
74898

Contents

"Happy is he who like Ulysses has made
a glorious voyage."

(Joachim du Bellay from Les Regrets, 1559)

Dedication

To my mother who lived to be old
And my father who didn't
And to all the amazing older people who have touched my life

Approaching Sixty

When is the time that we realign our picture of ourselves and move from thinking of ourselves as young to thinking of ourselves as part of the older generation? There's no doubt that this transition occurs differently for each person. Often we may not notice the exact time until we can look back.

For me (looking back), I pinpoint that time as the days when my sixtieth birthday crept closer and closer. From that time on, I have experienced an internal shift—a shift in my own worldview. Turning sixty seemed to signify a huge change in how I looked at my life. I still looked ahead but began to know that I had already lived the larger portion of my life. It felt like time to take stock, time to ponder how I felt about my own aging and aging in general. How did it feel to think of myself as older?

The truth is, I've had a terrific reverence for and appreciation of older people for a long time. These feelings have been affirmed over and over in the past twenty years that I have worked with the elderly and their families. So the idea of joining their ranks has seemed like a privilege. Getting older carries with it the wonderful chance to continue one's growth. What a marvel that can be!

The specifics of my sixtieth birthday celebration seem particularly pertinent to my own way of moving out of middle age and into life as an older person. I tend to come on like gangbusters.

Because I love celebrating, I began to think of how I might want to mark my sixtieth. I considered some of the options: A trip with my husband and adult children? A party with close friends? It wasn't until we were on a canal trip in the south of France with two other couples that I found the answer to this question.

On our trip, we piloted our own boat along the beautiful Canal du Midi, often stopping to see the vineyards or charming towns along the way. We would tie up when evening came and spend the night moored to the bank. We had one very scary night when the mistral blew fiercely. All of a sudden, we were awakened by a huge change in the position of our boat. One of our mooring ropes had broken free, and we hung on by the other. Our boat was sitting sideways in the canal. It was pitch-black. It seemed like the middle of the night, but it was actually somewhere between four and five in the morning. We all got up out of our beds and worked together to let the wind blow the boat back around so we could fasten the ropes securely again.

Later that morning, the wind was still blowing, and the women in our party decided we would ride our bikes to a grocery store to replenish our supplies. I got on my bike and started up over the steep cement bridge, which spanned the canal. I realized I wasn't making any headway and that I really ought to get off my bike and walk. Too late! My bike and I came crashing down. I hit my head on the bridge with a resounding crack! We were all pretty concerned about me. Besides tremendous embarrassment at my own clumsiness, I worried whether I might have a concussion and whether I would need medical assistance. I got some of our precious ice (ice was in short supply, and we would ration it out for the all-important cocktail hour!) and held an ice pack to my head while my friends biked on through the terrible wind. Fortunately, I did not have a concussion and didn't even have a bad headache—just a big lump on my head!

The next morning, I awoke at 5:00 AM with a fantastic idea (that I felt came from that wallop on the head). I tried to wait for my husband to wake up but couldn't contain myself. I began whispering my idea to him. (The walls of the cabins in the boat were paper-thin.) My idea was to celebrate my sixtieth birthday by learning a piano concerto and playing it with a full orchestra. At that point, my birthday was approximately one year and nine months away.

The idea of playing a piano concerto was no mere fantasy. I have been a pianist since I was young and have studied piano all my life. So when we returned home from that canal trip, I began pursuing my goal with a focus and clarity that I'd never had before. I launched into the arduous practice routine that I would maintain until the event. I already knew whom I would need as my teacher and coach. I had studied piano with her in the past, and she was a performer herself. Not only could she guide me as I learned the notes (what a lot of notes there were), but she could also play the orchestra part with me to help me learn how the solo sounded with the orchestra.

It was somewhat like training for a marathon. I needed to be in tip-top physical and mental condition to pull it off. I wanted to eat right and exercise along with the mental challenge of learning the piece. The concerto I wanted to learn was by Robert Schumann. It's very romantic, and romantic fitted my temperament. Mozart seemed terribly exposed, and Beethoven and Brahms seemed out of my league. And I have always been fascinated by the story of Robert and Clara Schumann. He wrote his only piano concerto for his beloved wife. Their story is beautifully told in the book *Longing* by J. D. Landis.

I settled down and began to practice. Oddly enough, I decided to learn the end of the piece first. My thinking was that those notes would be the most rehearsed of all so that I would feel the most confident at the end. I remember sitting at my piano after playing the final chords and wondering how it would feel when I heard those chords with a full orchestra behind me.

Practicing the piano has always been a satisfying experience. You start out feeling like a beginner.

Learning the notes can be a tremendously tedious process. Also, to feel secure, I would need to memorize most of the piece even though I would have the score in front of me. So it all seemed pretty slow going. I set goals for myself like I'll learn five pages by such and such a date. Or I would try out the first movement by a certain time. It helped keep me focused and prevented me from bogging down with the enormity of my task. The best thing about practicing is when you look back over six months and see how far you've managed to come. And once you gain the mechanics of the piece (no small task when it came to learning the Schumann), it is then possible to focus on the music itself.

While I worked away at the piano, my husband acted as my unofficial "agent" in our search for an orchestra and performance space. After listening to various local orchestras, I felt incredibly lucky that the Arlington Symphony agreed to work with me. An additional plus was that they had just moved into a beautiful new hall that we felt would be perfect for my event.

We were in negotiations with the orchestra about the timing of my event when I heard the Schumann concerto on the radio. When it finished, the announcer said, "That was Robert Schumann's piano concerto, and we played it today because today is his birthday." The date was June 8, 2001. My sixtieth birthday would be June 17, 2002. I thought, *Wouldn't it be great to have my event on Schumann's birthday?* We signed a contract with the orchestra for a concert on June 8, 2002. The orchestra would play a piece on their own (I picked Rossini's overture *to La Cenerentola*), and I would play the Schumann concerto.

Now the heat was on. I knew my deadline. In the next months as I gradually worked through all three movements, I played the whole concerto through five times with my teacher playing the orchestra part. I needed to gain confidence with the material in front of an audience, so I staged crucial tryouts with friends and family acting as audiences.

My husband and I worked together on all the details. We sent out invitations, planned the reception for after the concert, designed and printed a program. Finally, the time came for my orchestra rehearsal. With the contract we had worked out, I only had one chance to rehearse with the orchestra before the performance. The concert was on a Saturday afternoon, and my only rehearsal was the Friday night before. Nighttime is not my best time to function. I concentrate and do my best work in the mornings. My sister joked that we should have the concert at 10:00 AM.

Needless to say, I was hugely anxious about how my rehearsal would go since I had no experience playing with an orchestra. I got onstage (with my trusty page turner), and my rehearsal began. Because of my lack of previous experience, I had no sense of what the sound of the piano with the orchestra would be. My only practice had been hearing how the orchestra part sounded played on a piano. The piano is a percussive instrument. Therefore, it can sound much louder than many of the instruments in the orchestra—particularly the strings. I found my playing much more exposed than I had anticipated. In my rehearsals with my teacher playing the orchestra part on a second piano, that second piano had often masked my mistakes. But it was not the case when it came to strings versus the solo piano. The other big challenge was that the Schumann concerto is devilish in that, in both the first and third movements, the composer had written the same passages but in different keys. During the rehearsal, the conductor would instruct that we would start on measure "so-and-so," and I constantly mixed up which key I was in, causing us to have to stop and begin again. It was excruciating. We finally got through the whole work, and there was a break. I tried to relax, but my stomach was in knots. I felt completely drained and exhausted and worried. Several members of the orchestra came over to me and said encouraging things, but I could hardly hear their much-needed support.

When the break ended, the conductor said, "Donna, now we'll run the whole thing without stopping."

I looked at her thinking, *You've got to be kidding*. I was sure I couldn't manage to muster up the energy to get through it again.

She said, "I know you're exhausted, but you need to *know* that you can get through it when you're not at your best."

I felt not only was I not at my best; I was truly at my worst. There I was, drained from my first experience ever of playing the Schumann concerto with a real live orchestra, and here was the conductor calling on me to do it again, this time without stops. "It's crucial that you can prove to yourself that you can do this now when you are exhausted. It will sustain you for the real performance," she assured me. So I sat back down at the piano.

Somehow, I did make it through without a serious hiccup. That night, when I finally got to bed, I looked over at my husband and saw a most haggard face. He had really gone through it too. Surprisingly, with the performance looming on the next day, I slept like a baby.

The day of the concert dawned sunny and beautiful. I remembered the conductor's words and began to think that she had amazing wisdom. I realized that I had played the whole concerto with very little energy. Surely I would succeed today. The concert was scheduled for three o'clock. The whole morning, I stayed in a sort of "zone." I remember feeling protected by a kind of bubble around me that allowed me to observe what was going on but kept me in my own space. I spent a brief time at the piano to keep the music fresh in my mind.

We set off for the performance hall with plenty of time for me to get dressed and prepare. (Unbeknownst to me, ninety-four thousand Girl Scouts were gathering in the mall in downtown D.C. that day. They presented a monumental traffic obstacle to many of my family and friends. One of my sisters made it to the hall just as I walked onstage! Thankfully, I knew nothing about any of that.) We arrived without incident, and I went backstage. My teacher had coached me to stay well away from people so that I could keep my concentration. I went to a room offstage to get dressed and do my makeup. My husband and children acted as hosts for our guests. People important to me began to gather. All my family (children, spouses, brothers and sisters and their spouses), close friends and friends of close friends, high school friends, professional friends, and some of my elderly clients came.

Three o'clock came. Still, the concert didn't begin. The waiting backstage was breathtaking. I remember drawing in deep breaths to try to stay calm. My teacher (who was my page turner) was backstage with me. We could hear the orchestra warming up. She remarked that that sound always made her the most nervous when she waited to perform. At about three ten, the orchestra played the overture to *La Cenerentola* (or Cinderella). When they finished, the stage director told us to come and wait immediately offstage while the piano was put in place. I remember looking out to the stage and feeling again in that special "zone." I wasn't shaking with anxiety. I held myself together. Still, underneath was a deep, lurking fear.

Then they cued us to walk on. The audience applauded; I bowed and sat down. I looked up at the conductor. She cued the orchestra, and with a resounding orchestral chord, we were launched. Luckily for me, Schumann starts the piano part immediately, so there was no more waiting.

What to say about the playing experience? I did stay in that zone of concentration. I certainly missed some notes, but they were not important to the overall performance. If I lost my place at all, my teacher would discreetly point to the correct measure in the music. I don't think the audience noticed. My husband (who knew the piece about as well as I did) certainly noticed. It's the third movement that is the most challenging. I got through the first two movements (including the cadenza in the first movement) with no real mishaps. However, in the third movement, I had a terrible lapse and lost my place. I could keep the notes in my left hand going but could not find how to come back in for the right-hand part. (My conductor had advised me not to try to get back in but to wait and enter when I felt certain of where I was.) During this terrifying space of time, my teacher was pointing to measure after measure, trying to help me. (My husband said later that it looked like she was tracking a bug!) In the nick of time, I gathered my wits and reentered just as a few bars of piano solo were required. I was able to go on and restore my concentration after that. The concerto surged to its dramatic climax. The conductor had been right. Because I had managed to play the concerto when I was at my worst, I was able to give the performance of my life.

My friends and family applauded, whistled, and cheered. My husband came onstage with flowers for me, and the clapping went on. Finally, the conductor spoke some very complimentary words and turned to the audience and said, "Now let's sing to her as she has been singing to us." The orchestra played "Happy Birthday," and the whole audience sang to me. People cried, especially me. The most amazing positive energy came toward me in the hall—flowing from the audience in front of me and from the orchestra behind me. I'll never forget it. Even today when I listen to the CD, I can feel the power of it. I still cry.

I carry the thrill of that day with me now. It's a touchstone and a demarcation for me. Before the time of "my concerto," I did not think of myself as old or senior. It's hard to pinpoint exactly when this transition transpired, but it was happening during those months that I was practicing my concerto. This change in thinking can be triggered in any number of ways: by the death or disability of one's parents, noticing that one's knees don't behave as they used to, discovering that the young girl who used to babysit for you is married and has children of her own. Whatever the prompt for me, I realized that I made an internal shift that caused me to think about my older status. The more I thought about it, the more I began to revel in the idea of my older self.

Open-Mindedness

If we hope to look at our aging as a kind of thrilling adventure, we must examine how willing we are to maintain an open mind. The benefits of keeping our minds open as we get older and older are crucial. While aging may narrow our lives in some respects, the need for receptive, open minds increases as we move toward old age. Only with open minds can we keep ourselves ready to embrace new ideas, form new relationships, take into account new technology, and allow ourselves new responses to life's new challenges.

Consider the alternative or the opposite of openness. We come up with descriptive words like *closed, rigid,* or *blocked.* Closed-mindedness shuts off our chances to see alternatives. Without an open mind, we deny ourselves the ability to entertain and consider all the novel and different scenarios that could be available to us. A truly open mind allows possibilities that we haven't even thought of. If we accept that all our life experiences affect our thinking and attitudes, then it's impossible to fully predict how we'll feel about something in the future. We don't yet know what experiences await us or how they can dramatically change how we currently feel.

Two stories from my psychotherapy practice demonstrate how open-mindedness (or the lack of it) can affect our lives as we age.

Rose

I first met Rose when she came to one of my therapy through music sessions at her assisted-living facility. She was a diminutive lady physically, but I soon learned about her unique personal strength and power. From the beginning, she exhibited an amazing openness.

She had moved to the Washington, D.C., area to be near her daughter and granddaughters. Although she readily admitted that moving out of her lifetime home had been extremely hard, she entered her new living situation with an open mind and a readiness to make a success of it. From the moment of our first encounter, she participated in my group music sessions with great energy and enthusiasm. Her open, friendly manner infected everyone around her. She soon knew the names of all her fellow residents. If I forgot someone's name, I would quietly ask for her help. When the group joined together to sing, she sang with an enchanting gusto—openmouthed and joyous.

Rose's magnetic personality drew people to her, and she forged strong connections with the staff and the residents. I felt an unusually deep, inexplicable bond with her—an affinity that I felt compelled to reveal to her. When we had that conversation, she smiled knowingly. She seemed to comprehend the intensity of my feelings. I was so moved that I found myself close to tears. Till the sad day of her death, all of us who knew Rose were profoundly touched by her wonderful, open exuberance. In her last years of life, she brightened all the lives around her.

Jen

Jen is a woman in her seventies. She and her partner have been together for over forty years. I became involved in Jen's case at the time her partner was feeling the burden of maintaining their big (and very old) house. Her partner was starting to entertain ideas of different living possibilities for them. Jen was pretty adamant about wanting to stay put and wasn't the least bit open to thinking about alternatives. She was not receptive to the idea of therapy either, but reluctantly agreed to a few joint sessions.

During our sessions, Jen was very strong in her opinions and spoke with authority on just about any topic that came up. She felt she knew what was best and held on rigidly to her own view of how she and her partner should handle things. She seemed unable to expand her scope to see other sides of the issues that arose.

Right in the midst of the time that I was working with Jen, she was diagnosed with serious heart blockages and ultimately had massive open-heart surgery. Interestingly, when I saw her after her recovery, she appeared softer and more pliable and easier to approach. It seemed that the surgery had exposed some of her vulnerability. I was hopeful we might progress in the therapy.

Yet over time, she reverted to her former self and now behaves very much as she did before the surgery—resistant, implacable, and unmovable. She continues to have serious health issues including depression. She still refuses to consider a change in living status that might benefit her and relieve the strain on her partner. Her partner complains that Jen is often angry about her condition and rails against getting older. Jen's inability to find ways to stay open to new possibilities is hampering her capacity to cope with her own aging and keeps her stuck in negative thinking. If she could open her mind and begin to see beyond her own narrow vision, she might be able to find new ways to adapt to, and ease, the challenges she faces as she ages. Her own lack of openness contributes to her dissatisfaction and negative thinking.

These two stories illustrate differing mental states we can bring to some of the life choices we encounter as we age. Let's look at the issue of openness: Rose walked into a new life open to new experiences and open to those people she encountered while Jen resisted fiercely the changes that occurred in her life and could not seem to allow new ideas to enter into her way of thinking. The end of Rose's life was filled with deep bonds and true affection and giving to others while Jen struggles with her own anger and frustration.

It is likely that Rose and Jen did not know in advance how they might behave when faced with experiences such as serious health problems or necessary changes in living arrangements. It is hard to envision our own futures. Of course, we make plans. But we cannot know *now* what twists and turns our lives will take. If we can develop this capacity for openness now, as "younger" old persons, we can use this approach to help us to deal with any challenges that aging may bring.

What might hamper us in our quest for an open mind?

While we may begin to see the value of staying open in our thinking, there are always potential pitfalls that can undercut our ability to remain open. One of the most obvious would be if we have a tendency to think and speak in absolutes. If we find ourselves regularly using words like *never, can't,* or *won't,* we have probably developed some habits that are closing our minds to other possibilities. Absolutes stop us and keep us stuck. While we may honestly believe that there are no other ways to see a certain issue, in fact, there are always a multitude of possibilities. Being absolutely sure about something closes the door to keeping open to things new or different down the line.

Feeling certain in the present does not give us the opportunity to know how our ongoing experiences may shape our thinking. All of us want to be free to grow and change. It's the way to stay feeling most alive.

The whole notion of judging is another factor that can stand in the way of open thinking. Harsh *self*-judgment can seriously hinder us in our efforts to remain open in our thinking about ourselves. We may decide that we have negative qualities and shut our minds to other ways to view ourselves. In addition, there's the factor of allowing other people's judgments to restrict our ability to let our minds roam free. Too much judging stops the imaginative process.

There's also the possibility that we have cluttered our minds with old resentments or old hurts. Hanging on to a lot of negative baggage may not leave space in our minds—space that would allow the *new* to enter. This is important when it comes to relationships. We need to stay open not only for shifts in ourselves but also for allowing others to grow and change. One area that comes to my mind when I think about allowing others to grow and change is when I consider my relationships with my grown children and in-laws. While they are certainly adults with huge adult responsibilities, they are relatively new to life's journey. Their own aging will no doubt change their perspectives just as my own has changed mine.

A story about my relationship with my mother-in-law illuminates the value of keeping ourselves open to the possibilities of change in our attitudes. When I was first married, I very much wanted to please my mother-in-law and be the kind of daughter-in-law she desired. My mother-in-law was an ultimate homemaker and had a wide range of interests and talents, including gardening and sewing and church activities. She also was an avid reader. Her primary values included the importance of education and making the best possible home for her family. She did not choose to work outside her home. I originally thought that life as a homemaker would be what I would want as well. As my own family grew (we had three children very close together), I realized that I desperately craved something outside my family to fulfill me. It was the height of the women's movement. Many women were looking beyond the homemaker role. I struggled with my conflicting feelings about whether it was OK to stray outside my role of wife and mother. My own values (and those of my mother-in-law) tugged at my choices. In spite of those conflicting feelings, I decided to pursue a career along with maintaining my role as mother and homemaker. I sensed disapproval from my mother-in-law. She would tell me about Sally, a young woman who was her friend. Sally stayed at home and took care of her children.

Over the years, I became more comfortable with my life's path and more secure with my choices. In turn, my mother-in-law seemed to grow more approving. She began to see me for who I was and seemed to accept me for myself rather than some preconceived notion of daughter-in-law. I'm glad we were both able to be open-minded and allow the changes in each of us to occur naturally. She lived into her eighties, allowing our relationship to morph into a wonderful closeness and intimacy. I still treasure my memories of her.

How can open-mindedness benefit us as we age?

Let's assume for the moment that we *want* to be more open-minded and take a look at how this quality can be a huge factor as we age. If we are willing to allow the new, it is difficult to stay stuck with the old. Openness can go a long way in reducing our anxiety about the future challenges of aging.

With the stories of Rose and Jen as guides, we will address the following four issues that may weigh on the minds of those of us "younger older people" as we look ahead.

1. Health
2. Mobility
3. Living arrangements
4. Relationships

Health

It's likely that, for most of us, the issue of our health may be at the top of the list of our concerns. Those of us who have begun considering aging issues already have far more information about maintaining good health than the generation before us. We know about the benefits of eating right and exercise to keep ourselves as fit as possible. We even know ways to keep our minds active and alert.

Still, however diligent we are, it is not possible to completely halt the impact of our own advancing age. We are living creatures, and like all living creatures, we will ultimately die. So how can open-mindedness help us if we live to be old and our bodies deteriorate?

There may be a number of innovative devices, remedies, or treatments that have not been discovered yet that can ease us in old age. Just look back twenty years, and it is easy to see changes that have affected the elderly. Twenty years ago, having a knee replacement was rather innovative and somewhat risky. Today, that procedure has been refined and is offered to older and older patients. The same goes for hips. Hip replacements are now virtually routine, and breaking one's hip is not the disabling condition it used to be. If we look ahead with open minds, we can view our own health issues with all sorts of possibilities.

Mobility

If we remain open-minded about our mobility, we may be surprised at what may be available to us. Over the past twenty years in my own work with older people, I have observed all sorts of new devices that have greatly contributed to their quality of life and independence. Things such as motorized scooters and wheelchairs are becoming common. One of my clients who had Lou Gehrig's disease found that having a scooter allowed her to move about on her own in her home. Without it, she would have been bedridden. A friend uses a scooter to maneuver around the grounds of her retirement facility, reducing her dependence on her partner to chauffeur her. Now she has much more choice about her own schedule. For others, elevators are routinely being installed in all kinds of houses, even beach houses.

Besides the issue of our own physical mobility, being able to drive a car is a major concern for most older people. In my experience with older clients, giving up driving is one of the hardest choices an older person faces. What new developments in the cars themselves may be in store for us? My friend has a car that beeps to let him know if he's getting too close to another object, and there are cars that can parallel-park themselves. Twenty years from now, cars may basically drive themselves. But say we do need to give up driving at some point. Most group living arrangements provide transportation. Hiring drivers is an option. And there are certainly solutions out there that haven't been thought up yet.

Living Arrangements

What will be our living choices as we get older? This question may provoke a certain amount of anxiety. What if we grow tired of maintaining that big house? What if arthritis limits our ability to run up and down the stairs? What if we are widowed and no longer want all the reminders of a shared living space? Again, the options and choices for us in the future will no doubt be varied and new. I have been amazed at the change in residential choices for older people in the twenty years I've been working with this population. It used to be that older people could choose to either live in their own homes, live with a family member, or live in some kind of nursing or care home. Nowadays there is a wide range of communal living arrangements for older people. Retirement facilities for independent living are booming and offer almost all services to their residents.

There is the option of assisted living that gives some assistance to residents who don't need nursing care. Nursing homes offer different levels of care depending on the needs of the patient. For those older people who still choose to live in their own homes, home-care options have also grown. And then there will be new living arrangements that haven't been thought of yet. The baby boomer generation is a massive, informed, creative group that will surely come up with new living styles—arrangements like friends combining resources to live together.

Relationships

Let's consider the area of relationships and how keeping an open mind can be so important. Living to be old carries with it the obvious potential for loss. Loss of significant people in our lives is something we will all face if we live into our eighties or nineties. Having an open mind leaves us willing to consider new connections as we age. New people in our lives can be a major source of emotional nourishment and stimulation. I'm thinking of my mother's openness to new relationships when she moved into a retirement home. She became very close to the lady across the hall. Esther was older than my mother (a fact in which she took pride). My mother found herself beginning to keep an eye on Esther. She was someone for my mother to care about. Mother would knock on Esther's door at mealtimes to make sure she got down to dinner. This new friendship provided a lovely connection for my mother and contributed greatly to her enjoyment and satisfaction in her new living environment.

Along with thinking about new relationships, we can consider our willingness to be open to new ways to think about and interact with our longtime relationships. Relationships with spouses, parents, adult children, and siblings and friendships may offer surprising opportunities for renewal and change if we aren't stuck in our thinking.

Sibling relationships are long-term connections that call upon us to be open to adjusting our thinking. Old patterns sometimes die hard, but as we age, staying open in thinking about our siblings is a requirement that will allow those relationships to change and grow. As a younger sister in my family, it has taken awhile for me to feel on a more equal footing with my older siblings. Take the case of my oldest sister (who is nine years older than I). When we were growing up, she seemed more of an adult to me than simply another child in the family. In some ways, I guess I was even a little intimidated by her. She was quite the achiever in high school, and I thought she even looked a bit like a movie star. I remember being a gawky preadolescent at her wedding, and in the early days of her marriage, we didn't really overlap much. Eventually, I finished college and focused on my own married life in California while she continued living in Kansas City where we had grown up.

After some years passed and I had moved East, I made a visit to Kansas City to see my mother and show off my new baby daughter. Coincidentally (I don't really believe in coincidences, by the way), my sister's husband chose that very time to announce that he was leaving her after fifteen years of marriage. My sister was devastated. As she tried to pick up the pieces of her life, she followed me to my home in Washington, D.C., and spent some days gathering her wits and trying to figure out what to do. We both remember sitting around all day reading a Taylor Caldwell novel and taking breaks to take care of my young daughter. In those sad and difficult days for her, I remember assuming a kind of caretaker role. I wanted to do whatever I could to ease the pain she was going through. During that time so long ago, our former roles of older and younger sister blurred, and I felt us relating to each other in a different way. If we both had not been able to keep our minds open to a new way of relating, we would have missed an opportunity to deepen our relationship and know each other in a new way.

How Can We Keep Our Minds Open?

Let's examine some of the factors that can lead us to open our minds.

We'll consider the following four:

1. **Experiences** that afford us a new or different outlook.

2. **The perspective of time** that can alter how we think.
3. **New information** that broadens our picture of life.
4. **An active imagination** that allows us to entertain new thoughts.

1. **Experience** may be the most powerful tool we can employ in our search for an open mind. Whatever we have actually lived through is likely to stay with us and affect us most deeply. Experiences hold all the resources that we'll need to draw upon to enhance our mind's ability to change and shift. I'm thinking particularly of the painful or stressful experiences. They are the ones with the most potential for opening our eyes to a new point of view.

   A woman I know told me her story and how experience affected a change in her own thinking. She frequented a restaurant that was a popular place for older people, and many folks came into the restaurant on walkers and canes. She admitted to being turned off when she went there and felt some pity for the people she saw. Subsequently, she had a serious fall and injured her knee, which required painful physical therapy and which compelled her to use a cane for some time. The experience, she said, led her to a big change of heart in her feelings and thoughts about all those older people. It caused her to feel nothing but respect and admiration for the courage and valor of those elderly folks. *Look at them,* she thought. *They've gotten themselves up and out in spite of their limitations.*

It should not be difficult for any of us to recall events or circumstances that have had a powerful impact on our thinking. It might be a useful exercise to look back and note a time we experienced that we remember as hard. What was our thinking before the event? Did we notice a new or different take on it once we had moved through the pain? Were there lessons to be learned? Did the passage of time help us gain a new perspective?

2. **The perspective of time**. As I've aged, I've found that I use the perspective of time

more and more to help me open my mind to different ways to think. By the perspective of time, I mean getting some distance past an event or interaction and looking back. This method can work in the short run or over the long haul. One can gain new insights into events long past. I find this tactic especially useful in opening my mind to new ways to view a past interaction—especially an interaction that felt painful at the time. By allowing time to pass, the pain invariably begins to subside and new understanding can drift into my thinking. Then we can focus less on our pain and delve into discovering different ways to interpret what transpired.

A friend of mine used this view to gain a clearer understanding about her mother, whom I'll call Fran. In the years after my friend's father died, Fran was driving and quite active. But as time passed, she became more reclusive and ventured out of her apartment less and less. She developed severe memory problems and needed assistance to remain in her apartment but adamantly refused most help. My friend felt strongly that Fran would benefit by moving to some sort of communal living. Aside from my friend's grave concerns about Fran's safety, she worried about her mother's aloneness and lack of social contact. Fran professed that she was fine on her own. She said she liked her own company and would not budge. Finally, Fran had an episode that involved her inability to walk, and she was hospitalized. My friend (who had allowed her mother maximum independence at the cost of her own anxiety about her mother being at risk) took the opportunity to move Fran into a nursing home and a safer environment. What time revealed to my friend is that during those last years when Fran left her apartment less and less, it may have been her own way to cope with her diminished memory. If she chose not to interact socially, she might be able to manage. It could have been that Fran was not particularly lonely and did not wish for more company. Indeed, she appeared to be quite content on her own in her apartment. Now that she lives in the nursing home, she does attend some activities, but she continues to seem comfortable with her own company. Only by allowing time to pass did my friend's mind open to a new way to view her mother.

There's the old saying, "Time heals all wounds." I'm not sure that it can heal everything, but the passage of time does allow for new thoughts and ideas and information to enter our minds and affect our thinking.

3. **Acquiring new information.** All through life, we are constantly exposed to new information. Especially today, in the age of the Internet, we have tremendous access to information. As we take in new facts and ideas from the endless resources around us, we are training our minds to accept new ways to conceptualize. We receive information in so many ways—through the arts, through reading, through the Web, through interacting with others, through travel, through work—just by living. It's all potential fodder for keeping our minds open.

4. **An active imagination.** We do not want to underestimate the power of our imaginations

as an aid in developing an open mind. In the practice of psychotherapy, we often say that if clients cannot *imagine* a different behavior or a different outcome in their lives, they are far less likely to be successful in *creating change* for themselves. Our imaginations are always available to us. Practicing using them can be enormously helpful. We can practice by imagining different scenarios for ourselves in our minds. Sometimes when I'm reading fiction, I try to imagine myself behaving like some of the characters—particularly characters whose lives are so different from mine. I say to myself, "Could I live like that?" Whatever I answer, I've allowed my mind to entertain a different idea of how to live. It's really an easy exercise, and I employ it regularly. I use it in my thinking about possibilities in relationships, in thinking sometimes outrageous thoughts, or imagining myself in completely different circumstances than my own. Years ago, I had a great opportunity to learn about the power of the imagination. I enrolled in a course called Creative Imagination

Methods, a nine-month course designed to help us access the amazing resource of our imaginations. The teacher had designed a vast number of exercises, games, and experiences that worked to open our minds. One I remember was called Oracles and Seekers. We each had the opportunity to be an oracle or a seeker. The seeker went to the oracle with an open-ended kind of question. Anything the oracle offered in the way of an answer was correct. There was no right or wrong answer. I can remember feeling the relief of not judging myself as I played the part of the oracle. If I trusted that whatever I said really was the answer, I began to feel truly wise. If we allow our minds to be free to entertain whatever floats in, we are open to all our imaginative power. That little exercise has had a great impact on my own approach to being open to possibilities. I maintain that there are *always* possibilities if we can keep our minds ready to consider them. This concept has proved extremely useful when I'm working with psychotherapy clients who declare they have no options.

Keeping our minds open is paramount as we age. With open minds, we will not be stuck in a world created by prejudging what our own aging experiences might be. In fact, there can be no way for us to know the unknown. In one of the focus groups I led before I started writing this book, one woman said, "I live my life knowing that anything can happen." True—we live knowing anything is possible. It is how we keep our minds open.

Most of us would agree that things have changed a lot in the past twenty years. Twenty more years of living can make quite a difference in what we may think or how we feel. We need to be open to what our experiences can teach us. However we choose to develop an openness in our thinking, there is no doubt that it can contribute to a more satisfying older age.

Coping with Change

As Mark Twain commented, "I'm all for progress; it's change I can't stand!" I doubt that anyone would argue with the fact that change is the one constant in life. And while we may agree with Mark Twain that we want to "progress" through life, how we feel about change and the transitions we may face may not be so easy or so clear. Whatever our attitudes toward change may be, change is inevitable. Some changes will be our choice, and some changes will occur, whether we like it or not. Time passes, and we realize that life is moving on.

Examining our attitudes toward change can be a key factor in predicting how well prepared we are to adapt to the changes that, we know with certainty, will come with aging. Determining what our strategies have been for coping with major changes in our lives can be a vital step in helping us age with confidence and reduce our fear.

Each of us, every day, experiences many examples of change—changes in relationships, changes in our bodies, changes in small things like our walking route or the way we do our hair. We can choose to look at these moments as opportunities to aid us in self-assessment. We can take the moment to ask ourselves the following:

How do I feel when change is occurring?

- Do I find it disorienting?
- Do I welcome variety?
- Do I feel scared or excited or possibly both?
- Do I look for ways to keep the status quo?
- Do I want to hang on to the familiar?
- Do I even notice that change is happening, or do I prefer to deny it?

Why is it important to have some idea about how we feel about change? This knowledge can prepare us for the future. Many of the changes we will encounter as we age will not be changes we choose. If we can see today that change *will* happen and find ways to gain some acceptance of this fact, then it will certainly ease our way down the road.

While some of the changes of aging will not be in our control, our feelings and attitudes *are* within our control if we have taken the time and made the effort to know ourselves and discover where those feelings and attitudes come from. Discovering the origins of our feelings takes a good bit of self-examination. For me, it is a lifelong process. Some may manage this exercise solely on their own. Others of us may need a therapist to assist us in this task. Whatever strategy we use, it is important to make ourselves aware of our feelings and attitudes toward change. Using that information can enlighten us about how we might feel when faced with unanticipated changes. If during this self-examination we find that we have a strong resistance to change, then we will need to look for ways to adapt and break through it. A persistent resistance to change will likely contribute to frustration and anger as we age and impede our ability to deal successfully with the challenges aging may bring.

For those of us who are already in our sixties or older, it is likely that we have already experienced some of the changes thrust upon us by aging: changes such as bodies that do not behave like they did ten years ago, relationship changes that can be painful, losses that bring acute grief. These kinds of changes provide perfect opportunities for the self-assessment I am talking about. As we get a grip on how our attitudes and feelings toward change can aid or hamper us, we can move on and look at *how* exactly we deal with change.

Everyone is coping with change in one way or another. Each of us possesses our own individual *coping style* as we age, and consciously or unconsciously, we assemble distinct ways we react when confronted by change. At first, we tend to be shaped by our early family life and whatever coping styles we learned as young children. As we mature, we formulate a specific style that is unique to each of us. How can we determine what is our style to prepare for future changes in our lives? If we can own and claim what has already worked for us, it can give us confidence that our coping resources will be sufficient to meet future changes. If we look at how we have handled significant transitions like marriage, divorce, children, job change, moving, or serious illness, we may learn what our coping strategies are.

As we analyze how we have coped, it may help us to ask these questions:

> What are my behaviors when faced with major change?
> What do I do that helps me feel competent?
> If I feel fear, what helps me feel less anxious?
> Which behaviors contribute to my sinking into depression?
> What helps me keep myself together?
> Who are the people I can rely on?

As an example, I'm looking back at one of my own major life transitions and thinking about what it tells me about my own coping style. In my case, I'm considering the birth of my children some thirty years ago. This turned out to be not only a major transition for me but also a turning point in my life.

I was a pretty traditional girl. I went to the state university. I expected to get an education degree (so that if anything happened to my husband, I could always provide for my family), and then I expected I would marry and have a family and live happily ever after. In fact, that's about how it happened.

I met the man I wanted to marry while we were in college. We married after we graduated. I did teach school in the beginning of our marriage to support us. The "having children" part was a little more tricky. When I didn't get pregnant easily, we decided to adopt. We got our daughter when she was thirteen days old, and we soon began to feel like a family. I remember hanging up her little bootees on the clothesline and being so pleased! When she was around two, we adopted our son. Again we were thrilled, and I tried to adapt to the demands of two young ones. However, my adaptation period turned out to be much shorter than I could have imagined when our infant son was about three weeks old.

We had a huge Christmas party on a Saturday night. The next morning, I really felt ill. All day I couldn't really get back any energy at all. I remember sitting with a friend and tentatively broaching questions about how one feels if one is pregnant. I can still see the somewhat horrified look on her face. I went to the doctor, had the test, and of course, it turned out positive. Our third child, a son, was born eight months later.

This is when the "happily ever after part" began to get dicey! I felt more and more swamped by the demands of two babies and a three-year-old. I had my own bout with depression, which continues to make me extremely sympathetic to those who deal with chronic depression. (In my case, I think part of it was postpartum depression, but my doctor never offered that diagnosis. Somehow having an acceptable label would have helped.) I also suffered repeated migraines. I felt isolated at home and not very connected to the outside world. I remember feeling I needed to read *Time* magazine before going out to a dinner party in order to feel current and "interesting." I did have friends who were also home with small children, but they seemed mostly content. I felt dissatisfied and frustrated. I really had no conscious plan of how to change my situation.

In short, I did not feel that I was coping well at all. Partly, it was the disparity between what I thought would bring me huge life satisfaction (having a family and being a mother) and how dissatisfied I actually felt.

I then chose to find a challenge outside my home. I arranged babysitting for the children two days a week and volunteered at Common Cause, a large lobby working to control campaign financing. It was exciting to be in downtown Washington, D.C., and in the center of a political struggle. My volunteer job was field organizing, which connected me to people in my home state of Kansas. I even got a business trip to Kansas to work with Common Cause volunteers in the field. It was the beginning of my life outside my home, which ultimately led me to more education and a decision to make work a major part of my life.

As I look back now, I can find clues that help me define how I coped with that one transition. I can begin to answer those questions about what my behavior is, what makes me feel more competent, what makes me less anxious, and what helps me keep myself together.

I can now define my own coping style:

1. In that long-ago transition, I felt a tremendous *internal push to change my situation*. It really wasn't conscious at the time. That push is what drove me to make a change. I now see that I depend on that inner drive whenever I'm tackling a change. More and more I've learned to trust what my subconscious is trying to tell me. I've found that amazing things can bubble up.

2. When I found the going tough back then, I consulted a psychiatrist about my migraines. *Using outside professionals* to help me gain equilibrium and focus is another part of my coping style. A gifted psychotherapist has contributed greatly to my own inner knowledge and growth over the years. I know I will turn to outside help when I need it.
3. *Talking to others*—my friends, my husband, and my family were also part of how I coped all those years ago. Being able to express myself and get feedback from others is a specific strategy I use to help me clarify what is really going on in my head. Speaking out loud enables me to hear myself in a different way.
4. Back when the children were small, my husband and I managed to take some trips on our own. *Getting away geographically* is also a piece of how I manage to gain perspective. Somehow, being physically away gives me a chance to step back and find some objectivity in my thinking. This use of distance can be enormously helpful.

All of us can use a similar strategy to discover our own coping style. Take a major change in your life. Whatever you did and however you behaved, you lived through that difficult time. Even if you felt (as I did) that you were *not* coping all that well, you *did* cope. Now, with the advantage of age and experience, you can consider the questions, What did I do that sustained me in that past transition? What strengthened me? What people were most useful to me? What tended to drag me down? Did I need the support of others, or was solitude what I craved? You can extract and identify those actions that helped see you through. You can realize your own strategies for dealing with change. Then you will be able to see how to apply your unique coping style to other transitions.

Now that I have an idea of which strategies are helpful to me, I know I can apply them to any hard transitions that I may face as I age. For example, now when I'm facing a painful transition, I'm more than ready to seek outside professional help. By knowing my coping mechanisms, I can employ them any time.

When I hear of someone dealing with treatment choices after a diagnosis of cancer, I ponder what I might do if I were faced with a similar dilemma.

Knowing a little about how vulnerable, fragile, and terrified one must feel when facing a life-threatening illness, I feel quite certain that I would not be functioning anywhere near my strongest. Relying on trusted intimates to shore me up and help guide me would be part of my coping strategy. Because I have developed this coping style over many years as I've aged, I am more likely to trust my own instincts in a time of crisis.

I know that aging will confront me with all sorts of changes—some that I may choose (like a change in my living situation) and many that I will not choose, like the loss of loved ones, loss of vitality, or illness.

As we examine our own behaviors and coping styles, we may decide we want to change a specific way we have acted or reacted. An amazing supervisor I had in my first social work practicum suggested trying out outrageous behaviors to get an idea of what it might feel like to behave in another way. He gave an example that he had tried. When a Hare Krishna follower approached him in an airport to pin a flower on his lapel, he leaped back and shouted, "Get away from me." How often have we had this kind of response in our minds when we've felt intruded upon? Yet we rarely act on these thoughts. This was definitely *not* typical behavior for this mild, gentle man. Still, he decided to try something different in an arena where no one was hurt. I think of this example when I'm trying to make some change in my own behavior. I realize that I can go anywhere I wish in my thoughts. This seems to correlate to a therapy tool that, simply put, is *Act as if.* When clients are working in therapy on trying to change a behavior, they may first try just to *act as if* they are behaving in the new way. Over time, if they can continue with their acting, a change in their feelings may follow, and they will truly have moved into a new mode of behavior.

For example, a client may not be satisfied with the way he expresses anger in exchanges with a loved one. Working with a therapist, he will need to examine what's behind his feelings of discontent and discomfort. Then the client can begin to try to change his way of reacting. If he tends to be explosive, he may want to *act as if* he is calm and not be so reactive. Over time, he may actually begin to feel calmer and more objective. This concept may be why sometimes just *thinking* of doing something out of character is enough to open our minds to new possibilities.

I find that it's easiest to experiment with a new behavior if we approach it in a playful manner. Thinking up new responses to telemarketers might offer a chance to try out being a different person. Instead of our usual (and probably angry) response before we bang down the phone, we might engage the person in a chatty way. We could try asking him for his phone number!

Our coping strategies may emerge consciously or unconsciously. I am reminded of my friend's mother. Over the years, this dear woman became my friend too. As years had passed, she had lost more and more of her memory. She began to find conversations almost impossible because she could not retrieve the words as they flittered through her mind. One wonderful thing about this woman was her memory for songs and her ability to sing. She remembered most of the words to most of the songs of her era. She could be heard in the halls of her nursing home singing away. She maintained an identity as a person who sang and was greeted with smiles and warmth by staff and visitors to the home. She presented a positive face, one that reflected her generally upbeat approach to life. I thought, *It's hard to appear depressed if you're singing.*

Thinking of older people who cope positively with change reminds me of a wonderful article I read in the *Wall Street Journal* (November 11, 2006) about a woman named Anne Porter. She published her first volume of poetry when she was eighty-three. At the time of the *Journal* article, she was ninety-five and still writing. She draws from the changes in her aging mind and body, even the painful ones, to enrich her work. She suffers many of the frustrations of getting old such as needing a walker to get around and having to wear oversize glasses for failing eyes, and she admits to a certain amount of memory loss.

But Mrs. Porter somehow manages to derive inspiration from these setbacks. She discovered a ticket in her purse that said, "Keep This Ticket," but realized she had no idea what it was for or how it got there. That mysterious ticket inspired this lovely poem:

> I keep it carefully
> Because I'm old
> Which means
> I'll soon be leaving
> For another country

Where possibly
Some blinding-bright
Enormous angel
Will stop me
At the border

And ask
To see my ticket.

The number of stories about people coping with change seems endless to me. The older I get, the more things seem to be changing almost minute to minute. A dear friend suffered a stroke a couple of years ago. All of us who know her were stunned. With the miracle drug, which her son called "liquid plumber," she was able to quickly regain her speech and mobility. However, a second clot went to her optic nerve and greatly impaired her vision. The life of this amazing woman provides countless instances of how to cope with a dramatic change in one's life's circumstances. Over time, she has taught herself to navigate the nuances of public transportation, she has accepted offers from drivers, and she has relearned reading and numerous other facets of her daily life. What impresses me the most though is the internal shift that was required of her. My friend is known for how much she helps others. Her generous, giving persona is common knowledge in her community. After her stroke, she found herself in the position of needing constant help from others. How hard this must have been! She was always the giver and less the taker. Over time (even though she still tells me she hates it), she has learned to graciously receive. Truly surprising and marvelous!

While it's easy to see that change is happening all the time in our lives, what is not so easy is handling all those transitions. Grasping some idea of our own coping strategies, accepting change as an absolute part of life, and knowing that we *can* find ways to adapt our behavior when needed will stand us in good stead as we carry on.

REALIGNMENT

During the breakfast that launched the idea for this book, a friend and I mostly discussed the idea of impending retirement. The word *retirement* seems to me to be a dated choice for what this transition means today. Retiring can also mean heading for bed. Retirement seems mostly about ending something.

I like the idea that we are realigning. Realignment brings to mind the notion of a kind of repositioning, a shifting. It carries with it a sense of movement—moving away from one thing and toward something new. It used to be that when one turned sixty-five, it was time to retire—time to leave whatever our work was—collect our gold watch, and settle down into the golden years (whatever that meant!). That image is passé. It just doesn't fit today's sixty-five-year-olds a bit.

The people I know who are considering retiring do not do a lot of sitting around or settling down. They may decide to leave their professions, but they certainly expect life after work to continue to be vital, creative, and productive. I don't hear much about resting on one's laurels. People seem to be seeking new challenges and new definitions for themselves. They are engaged in realigning themselves to adapt to a new phase of life. Any of us who are currently in this phase or are approaching it will soon discover how much adjustment and "remodeling" is required of us.

A look at "realignment" requires some recognition and insight into what we previously aligned ourselves with. What are we shifting from? If we have stayed home, kept house, and reared a family, what new challenges are we looking for? If we have devoted ourselves to a profession, what is there beyond that work that we yearn to try? If we have felt our time constrained by a hectic job (whatever the job), how can we adjust to an easier, more open day? If we are in a relationship, what kind of impact will our realignment have on our partner?

These questions and others plagued my husband and me in the lead-up to his retirement from thirty years with his law firm. His career was a major source of challenge, creativity, and satisfaction for him. As with many of us, his identity was strongly linked to his work. What life would be like after he retired was a big unknown for him and for me. I had serious qualms about what our life might be like without that anchor of work for him. It was hard for me to imagine him without the mantle of work on his shoulders. Our story is one model for dealing with the issues most of us will likely face when approaching retirement.

Using his parents' example, we gave ourselves about five years to prepare mentally and financially for this dramatic transition. As far as the financial aspect was concerned, we did what most folks try to do: guessed what our needs would be. While financial issues are paramount (and there are numerous resources with advice on this topic), it was surprising that most of our difficult discussions focused not on money, but rather on emotional issues, personal space concerns, and day-to-day living together.

As the partner of the retiree, one of my chief fears centered around the use of our house. I have always worked from home and felt quite possessive about the house being *my* space. I expected that it would be quite difficult to begin sharing it. In numerous conversations, we thrashed this out together. We decided that my husband would create a completely self-sufficient home office for his use—separate computer, separate phone line, separate everything. We expected that we would each need a defined apartness.

I frankly can't remember all the discussions we had over the five-year period, but we did need plenty of lead time to address the complex issues that surround such a major life change. (A scary bout with melanoma—thankfully caught and successfully treated—prompted my husband to speed up the timing for his retirement.)

For most of us, one issue that looms large is how we'll use our time after retirement. Finding some kind of anchor or structure is one way to lessen our anxiety about this unknown. In my husband's case, he did some concrete preparation. Several years before his proposed retirement date, he tried teaching a course at a local university. He designed a course that fell under his own area of law practice and drew on the expertise he'd gained over the years. He then taught this course regularly in the spring semester in the years leading up to his retirement. The benefits were many and continue today. Besides giving him a ready answer to that question, what are you going to *do*? the course has forced him to keep current in his field. Added to that was the new challenge of teaching—a skill he wasn't sure he had. He surprised himself as he developed ways to stimulate and excite students. Taking on something new, either in retirement or in preparation for retirement, is one way to stay in the game and keep your mind active.

My husband also fits into that category of retirees who looked forward to having time for various pleasures—gardening, reading, house projects, etc.—which always took short shrift while he was working.

Retirement itself, it seems to me, is all about preparing yourself to plan for the concept of *not* planning. I guess that sounds like a paradox, but most happily retired people I know talk about the pleasure of having days free that they can structure however they wish. Before the fact though, thinking about all that open time can cause tremendous anxiety about a fearful unknown. Living a retired or realigned life is not something we can really understand until we're actually doing it. All through life, we are called upon to step into unknown places. We can choose how we step. We can go carefully and thoughtfully. We can analyze thoroughly. We can leap with confidence. We can go kicking and screaming. (Sometimes an employer decides for us that we must leave our work.) We can be excited or scared or both. We'll most likely act out this step according to our own personality style. Whatever our mode of behavior, we will call upon all those coping skills that we've amassed along life's way.

After my husband and I processed the concept for almost five years, the day of his retirement dawned, and we found ourselves trying out all the things we had tried to talk through. There was a delightful honeymoon period for about six months, and then life began to settle into a new pattern. We certainly experienced many a bump along the way. Living differently always requires us to adapt and change—not necessarily easy tasks.

Although I have a most helpful and considerate husband, he can go overboard at times. A little example of a big irritation was his attempts to "help" me. (Keep in mind I'd managed my workdays just fine for many years without him around.) He would remind me that I had phone messages and would even pick up my phone at times. Gentle hints that this was not acceptable and was intruding on my space didn't really work. After some serious, heated conversations, he got the message and now resists his urge to "help."

Living side by side in the house took some getting used to, that's for sure. For couples who have been together for a long time, one partner's retirement will lead to changes in living patterns that have set in over the years. Having my husband at home every day changed a number of long-established routines. He wanted to try his hand at doing more of the cooking. That seems like an acceptable idea, but it did require me to partially relinquish my provenance over this area of our life together. At first it was hard to give up what I viewed as mine. I liked doing the cooking and enjoyed the rewards of putting on a well-received meal. Having been in charge of the house and meals for over thirty years, I saw his advances into the kitchen as a major role shift. While part of me liked the idea of doing things differently, I have to admit I was also jealously guarding old patterns that were comfortable.

Over time though, we both began to see the advantage of changing roles. I was still going out to work every day, and now he was the one at home. I came to appreciate his "homemaking," and he was much more able to get an idea of what my workday was like.

In an odd way, his retirement increased my awareness of all those long days that he had put in over the years. I guess it might have been that I noticed the contrast to his much more relaxed life after retirement.

For us, all the *before* discussions made the actual act of retirement much easier. These discussions involved hashing out what each of our worries and concerns were. We ran through various possible scenarios and discussed how we felt and what seemed to cause our anxiety. I certainly leaned on my therapist to help me sort out my own feelings of anxiety. I think I had a serious fear that my husband might feel adrift without his work. Work had played such a hugely important part in his life for so much of our life together. Over time, I came to realize how ready for a change he was, and I gradually relaxed about this issue.

As my husband says now, "I really never looked back." This thought was echoed by a friend of mine. She said she never looked back. She thought it was because she was doing exactly what she wanted to do. She had shaped the life that she had hoped for after work. When we talked about this, she was quite clear that she had a pretty good idea of what she really loved doing (including gardening, cooking, time with family and friends) before she ever left her job. It's this piece of the realignment picture that most of us struggle with the most, and I can see why it's so hard. If we no longer spend long hours working, we are faced with the task of assessing just exactly how we want to use those available hours. What is it that we really love? Do we have activities that we feel passionate about? If so, how can we create the life after work that truly works for us? Can we risk possible failure in trying something completely out of our realm of expertise?

All of this requires a great deal of gentleness with ourselves. Can we seek without really knowing exactly what it is we're seeking? Can we be in our "found" time without harsh judgments about its use? Do we have a tendency to feel guilty when we choose to spend time on ourselves? Living in this new time "after work" will most likely be a way of experiencing time that we've never had before. It can be one of the joys and frustrations of the realigned life.

My husband went into his realignment with some specific projects that he hoped to accomplish in addition to teaching—activities that would offer a focus and purpose. He designed and created a back garden in our small backyard. He finished off our basement into a neat little apartment. And he joined me in what I now think of as my concerto project.

While I spent time at the piano learning all those notes, my husband acted as my agent as we threaded our way through the complexity of attempting such an event. He helped find the orchestra, worked on the contract with it, and attended to many of the numerous practical details involved. This collaboration, which was a focus of creative energy for both of us, helped forge the togetherness that had become part of his retirement. Some sort of cooperative project may help couples ease into a change. It could be shared grandparenting, building their own retirement home, playing golf together, planning trips, and traveling together—any number of creative and satisfying "togethernesses."

Our retirement experience exemplifies only one way to approach the transition of retirement. Not being bound by work can allow us to pursue some long-forgotten passion or just find out what it feels like to live moment to moment. We all will have our own timetables. Without the outside pressure and deadlines of work, we can select and discard options. Yet all that choosing may feel daunting. Practicing beforehand is a good idea, but it's difficult when we are bound by strict work hours and high-pressure schedules. Vacations and weekends may be the closest we come to knowing what it might be like. We can take a look at vacations and weekends and ask ourselves, How easy is it for us to have unscheduled time? Is it relaxing or anxiety-making to have an unplanned day? What do we choose?

The hope is that realignment can offer us opportunities to try out new behaviors. We may discover, for example, what it's like *not* to plan so much. One of my sisters worked full-time raising six children as well as working full-time in an outside-the-home job. When she retired, she devoted some time to her love of gardening and being in her yard. But she also found herself lazing in some of her days—watching videos and planning nothing. This is a woman who pushed herself tremendously during all those working years. She was allowing herself afterward a time to *breathe*.

However we prepare for this major change will be peculiarly unique to our own personality. For some, intensive research and an accumulation of facts can make something new more comfortable. Others may informally "interview" friends who are already retired to get an idea of what has worked for them. Others may try out one new challenge before retirement to see how they like it as my husband did with his teaching.

Whatever our strategy turns out to be, we may find it useful to gain some appreciation of exactly what we are most apprehensive about. Is it the issue of not knowing the answer to the question, what are you going to do? Is it the fear of the lack of daily structure? Is it worries about how our identity may change without our work persona? Is it deep concern about financial security? If we can name our fears, we are already one step toward dealing with them. If we can admit to ourselves what frightens us, then it is more likely that those coping mechanisms, which we have developed, will kick in—either consciously or unconsciously.

Realignment is just one of the challenges we'll face in our journey toward old age. Because we've already faced many a life challenge by the time we consider realignment, I'm convinced we already have within us the skills to manage this huge change without paralyzing fear.

Relationships That Age Well

When I think of clients, family, or friends who are happy in their skins and find delight in getting older, I'm aware that most of them put a high value on their connections to others. They thrive on their interactions with significant people in their lives. Their relationships demand their attention and energy and provide them with food for their souls. When I say *relationship*, I think of the whole gamut of relationship possibilities. Relationships such as parents and children, partners and spouses, friends, and any intimate personal connection we make with another person. I'm thinking of those ties we have to people who are so necessary in our lives that we'd have trouble imagining what our life would be without them.

If relationships are so crucial to us, we want relationships that will age well. What are the ingredients of such a relationship? We all may have our varied definitions. Mine turned out to be a mix of ingredients.

One of the most vital aspects of any lasting relationship is that it allows participants to be open and candid, to trust each other and assure both parties the freedom to be oneself with another person. It would be extremely constraining to maintain a connection to another person over many years and yet not be able to relax enough to be oneself. Not only do we need to be able to *be* ourselves, but we also need to have our *selves* accepted and respected. In the process, we need to achieve some confidence about our true selves. I expect to continue adding information and broadening my picture of myself until the day I die. Now that I am in that country of elders, I find that I do possess a better idea of who I am than I did when I was younger.

When I ponder my relationships, it's the connections with people who feel secure about themselves that I experience as the most intimate, nourishing, and satisfying. Long ago a young man taught me about this aspect of relationships. He was twenty-five years old when I met him. For the William Kapell International Piano Competition, we had offered our house (and my grand piano) to a contestant. We were matched with him, and for about a week, we had the divine pleasure of hearing this virtuoso pianist practice in our house.

One of the many attributes of this talented man was his own clarity about himself and who he was. When I asked him what he wanted (whether it was what to eat or what his goals and aspirations were), he not only knew what he wanted but was also able to articulate his wants and needs clearly and directly. I find this kind of honesty from another person a huge relief. It takes away that aspect of guessing what is really going on with him or her. One can trust so much more easily. As a result of this trust, we developed a rapport and closeness—a closeness based on an equal sharing of ourselves. After the competition, we had the privilege of attending his debut recital at the Lincoln Center in New York. We've stayed connected to him and have followed his career for many years. The essential trust and honesty established at the beginning of our friendship have continued and deepened.

In talking to my adult children about self-discovery, I've counseled that it often helps to know what we *don't* want. I think that we all have some sort of sifting process that, over the years, allows us to clarify to ourselves what our true desires are. When considering what I really want, one of my own rules about ambivalence is "When in doubt, don't!" Over and over, I've found that if I feel ambivalent about an option, I'm better-off not choosing it.

A mother-in-law/daughter-in-law story is illustrative. A friend was remembering the time her mother-in-law decided not to make any more overnight visits to D.C. It happened to be on a weekend when she and her husband and mother-in-law had enjoyed an exceptionally pleasurable few days together at their home in D.C., which even included attending a tennis match.

On the morning that her mother-in-law was leaving, my friend came back to the house after a walk. Her mother-in-law was sitting on the deck with sunglasses on, facing the sun. She appeared to be soaking up the September warmth. My friend said it was a singularly lovely image that remained with her always.

On that particular day, her mother-in-law announced that she would not be coming back on Christmas. As my friend drove her to her home in rural Virginia, she attempted to talk her out of the notion of no more visits. (She felt acute grief at the idea of losing her mother-in-law's presence at family gatherings.) As my friend later recounted the story, she knew that she wasn't making a dent in her mother-in-law's resolve to stay away. While her mother-in-law was never specific as to her reasons for such a decision, my friend guessed that the impetus might have come from two sources: her mother-in-law's concern for her own declining health and her desire not to be any kind of burden for her son and daughter-in-law. Her mother-in-law had almost taken a fall during her weekend stay, so the potential for future falls might have been on her mind.

Her mother-in-law stayed true to her word (and to herself). She did not return anymore. She ultimately did move to a nursing home in the D.C. area. While we may not fully understand another person's rationale for the choices she makes, perhaps the best we can do is respect her decision and allow her to remain true to herself.

The perspective of time has widened my friend's picture of that long-ago day when her mother-in-law sat on her deck. She recalls it with an awareness that her mother-in-law might have been storing up more than the sun's rays that morning. She seemed to be consciously absorbing the experience of what would be her last weekend visit with her son and daughter-in-law.

Relationships that age well not only accept others for who they are, but also for however they may change. For me, this takes continual vigilance. When one has known someone for thirty or forty years, there may be a tendency to start feeling like an authority on that other person. It's natural to presume this. After all, we've been connected for so long. Surely we *know*! The stunning part for me are realizations of how little I actually do know about a husband of forty-plus years, children I've known for thirty-some years, and longtime friends. To illustrate: in the late 90s, my husband was diagnosed as having a melanoma on his face. Fortunately, a dermatologist caught it early. Still, it was terribly scary going into the surgery. My husband had always had a kind of phobia about hospitals. His mother had a number of surgeries, and his memories of hospitals were painful. (When

I had an arthroscopic procedure, he admitted he almost fainted when he was with me as the nurse drew blood.) I was extremely worried about how he would manage his anxiety when the time for his surgery came. We drove to the hospital, and I was with him during the preparation. What I did not know until we were in the pre-op was all the thinking about his impending experience that he had done on his own. Instead of anxiety, I saw genuine calm and mental preparedness. He showed a side of himself I had not known in all our years together.

If you think about it, we have rather limited access to the extensive information available on someone else, particularly when we consider the other person's thought processes. Sometimes we may be confronted possibly very painfully with unexpected behavior from another party in a long-term relationship. These behavior surprises have the ability to throw us and discombobulate what appeared to be our usual pattern of relating. Allowing for these changes in the other person is one of the keys to having a long-term relationship that works.

Many of my friends and I have lost both of our parents. We talk about them and who they were. How well did we really know them? In most cases, parents and adult children live quite separate lives, often separated geographically. When I think about my mother, I realize it wasn't possible to know my mother's activities and thoughts—nor she to know mine—when she was in her 60s and I in my 30s (or at any time for that matter). She lived long enough for me to know her better, but looking back, I realize how much I did not know. We see only a part of the picture of another person.

Those of us who have become grandparents frequently wonder now about how our mothers viewed their own grandparenting. Did they discuss us and our child-rearing styles with their friends? Were they critical or accepting? Did they want to be more or less involved in our lives? We can use what we have known about our mothers to try to answer these questions, but we realize that it's hard to divine.

To construct a relationship with your parent (or child) that allows each of you to reveal the real you takes courage. All of us have parts of ourselves that are not known to those near and dear. We all have notions in our heads about the qualities a good mother or father should possess—and about the qualities we would want in a child. Good parent-child relationships require that both the parent and the child adjust their pictures of each other as they mature. As we become adult children to our aging parents, we should try to enlarge our perspective of our parents and attempt to see them more as people and somehow less as parents. This can allow us to drop some unfulfilled expectations we may have had of our parent.

If our parents live to be old, we may need to reverse roles and become their caretakers when we have had a lifetime to become accustomed to their caring for us. Our willingness to cultivate a more equal relationship may allow our parent to evolve as a person. This process can continue even after parents die. New information about these central people in our lives may emerge years after they are no longer with us.

At my mother's ninetieth birthday party, my sister had come across diaries that my father had kept at the time he was courting my mother. None of us knew of them before. My sister read brief excerpts at the celebration, and new glimpses of our father as a young man came to light. Especially endearing was his description of our mother as "keen." What a gift to learn more about this man who had died at the early age of fifty-seven.

As children we tend to assume that our parents are powerful and can keep us safe. Children deserve parental love. Childhood provides us with our working materials to shape our lives. These materials may be sorely lacking or generally proficient. Whatever we were given or deprived of merges into the self we make of ourselves as we age. When we attain a certain level of maturity and comfort with ourselves, we can reshape our pictures of our parents. Without a sense of self-worth, we are likely to have difficulty gauging our parents' evolution.

Sometimes an emergency can open up a child's eyes to vulnerability in a parent. I remember a camping trip with my parents and younger brother when I was about ten years old. We were going by motorboat at one point, carrying all our camping gear across a lake. We could hear a falls in the distance. The motor on the boat decided to conk out, and I can remember my father frantically trying to get it restarted. The falls got closer and closer, and I had such a clear sense of my father's fear. It was a defining moment for me. My strong, seemingly fearless father was afraid! Thankfully, he managed to restart the motor near the last second and get us safely away from the falls.

Just being able to see fear in a parent begins the process of a changing perception. With clients and adult children, I have often observed an adult child hanging on to perceived power and strength in an elderly parent long past the time the parent was capable of behaving powerfully or strongly. Opening our eyes to the vulnerability of our aging parents may take a good deal of growing up and inner strength. This can be especially true if our parents fiercely guard themselves from revealing any possible weaknesses.

There's no getting around the fact that a maturing parent-child relationship calls upon both sides to continually adjust their perceptions. For parents, it is also necessary to find ways to let go and to accept their children as functioning adults. While we want to acknowledge the wisdom we've gained in our own aging, we may want to remind ourselves that it was our own living through difficult or painful experiences that taught us the lessons. As parents it's natural to want to protect our children from hurt, danger, trauma—all that bad stuff. We hope to advise our children and help them sidestep the troubles and grief about which we have firsthand knowledge. But if we're really honest about it, it's our own trials by fire that may have forged our characters the most. So as parents, we may find ourselves biting our tongues or zipping our lips in order to allow our children to learn their own life lessons in their own way.

With a very old parent, adult-to-adult may seem to revert to a reverse parent-child relationship. Possible childish behavior in the parent may require caretaking responsibilities by adult children, but our aged parent is not a child with no former life.

Parenting children seems all about nurturing the child. But since all relationships are two-way, the child affects the relationship too. When a child moves into adulthood, one hopes for a gradual balancing in the relationship. As parents we hope to relate to our children more adult to adult. Achieving that kind of balance calls for a willingness on both sides to be open to self-examination and an ongoing reevaluation of what is working in the relationship and what may need to change.

I remember an issue with my mother that is a tiny example of a shift on her part to accepting me as an adult. We weren't living in the same city, so our chances to see my mother were mostly her visits to us. This was in part because she could more easily afford to travel to us than vice versa.

She liked to give gifts and spend money on us and would always want to take us out to dinner. This was, of course, a treat for us with our then-limited budget. Over time, however, we decided we wanted to pay for some of these dinners. (Were we growing up?) As I remember it, it took some convincing, but my mother ultimately did seem to understand this new dynamic. Certainly, money matters are an arena in which parents may need to shift out of parent mode and into a cutting of the apron strings to allow adult children to make it on their own financially. We all want to help, and help may, in fact, be appropriate. Still, it always seems like a balancing act to me—trying to weigh when to step in and when to step back.

In the case of parents and adult children, both sides will need to keep their antennae tuned to all the changes that may be going on. Adult children will no doubt want more and more autonomy and a respect for their adult lives. Aging parents may look for signs that their adult children have the ability to see them more as whole people with all that that means: people with vulnerabilities, strengths, and needs. It takes ongoing vigilance and commitment from both sides of any relationship for the relationship to stay alive and healthy.

A relationship that ages well cannot remain static very long. If the relationship is growing, it will continually change. That can be complicated when one acknowledges that one of the nicest things about a long relationship is that it's familiar and comfortable. It's about how to keep a relationship growing while getting more and more familiar and at ease with one another. How do people in satisfying long relationships manage to do that?

I'm sure the answers are as unique as the individuals in these kinds of relationships. Still, a lot of it comes down to how much growing is going on for each half of the relationship. We each do have a responsibility to ourselves to search for ways to grow, to maximize our talents, to live as fully as we can. Then, what we bring to a relationship is likely to be as vibrant as possible. Sometimes, of course, over the life of any relationship, the challenge may be that the growth spurts for both participants do not follow the same time line or stay in balance. People in long relationships tend to work on staying sensitive to what is transpiring in each other's life until some sort of equilibrium can return.

Let's look at potential pitfalls in the whole aging process of a relationship. A big danger in my mind is the assumptions we may make about each other.

As we're getting comfortable and familiar with another person over many years, we can fall into a sort of ESP mode and intuit a lot about the other person's reactions, feelings, facial expressions—you name it, we've become accustomed to it. While this can be part of the ease of the relationship, it might also lead to a kind of dulling of our awareness of the changes that might be occurring within the other person. Staying awake and alert to nuances and signals from the other person is a must if we hope to remain connected to that person over a long time.

This is not easy. Besides the day-to-day business of just living, there are tons of distractions for any of us that may contribute to a gradual lessening of our insight about a longtime partner. I have found that one of the biggest distractions for me is *myself*! I can get so focused on my own internal workings, issues, thoughts, traumas, or whatever that I may not keep my eyes and ears open to those who fit into my category of long-term, long-loved relationships. I may not notice the subtle, gradual changes in them. The others may not even be aware of some deep inner turmoil. Couples who engage in the effort of maintaining a relationship that remains satisfying for both parties over their lifetimes have some appreciation of the complexity and rewards involved.

But it's not only couple relationships that require this kind of active sensitivity to endure. Any long-term relationship (whatever its nature—couples, friendships, or the myriad possibilities in families) has the potential for those in the relationship to take each other for granted. And this can be deadly for the relationship.

Open channels of communication would appear to be a given in any relationship and certainly a requirement in one we want to last over time. Attention to *how* we communicate is probably as important as *what* it is that is being said. Have we become so used to the reactions and body language of our longtime other that we are not paying attention anymore? Do we feel we already know the answer to something we may ask? Are we very good at presuming the outcome of a conversation? Do we still care what message may be behind the other person's words? Are we still paying attention to facial and body cues? Do we get lost in the *words* sometimes and ignore what may be obvious signals of distress from the other person? These kinds of questions may help us look at ourselves and how our own behaviors can contribute to either keeping those vital lines of communication open and alive or how we may have a hand in a kind of shutdown. In a mother-child relationship, the mother is one sort of person as a new mother. She may or may not have confidence about her mothering skills. She may or may not be in a good place in her own life at the time. She may be very insightful and thoughtful about her mothering, or she may just wing it and muddle through the days. Whatever the description of the mother, she is changing, learning, growing as time passes. The same goes for baby. Baby arrives and gradually affects his or her world. Baby's own personality becomes more and more apparent and alters the relationship between mother and child.

Mothering skills must adapt as the child ages. This can be especially true in late life when an aged mother deals with her adult child and vice versa. What ingredients have gone into that mother-child relationship that will allow it to age well over the years? Have the mother and child been able to be clear with each other about their feelings over the years? Is there an underlying trust in the relationship and a belief that each is functioning as best as possible? Do they have an open pathway for the expression of affection? Are they willing to really listen and to hear each other? Answering these kinds of questions may assist us if we are called upon either to aid an aging parent or to find ways to relate with our own adult children as we become aged ourselves.

One friend pondered the possibility of some frank discussions with her adult children now that might prepare them (and her) for the possible future challenges of dealing with old age. I appropriated her idea, and we seize chances to bring up topics with our adult children about our futures as older parents—topics like how we might cope if one of us was diagnosed with Alzheimer's, how we feel about the idea of living in a nursing home, what living choices we might make after the sale of our house.

Siblings

For most of my elderly clients, sibling relationships seem to rate extremely high on their lists of important connections. Siblings are unique in that they alone have shared our earliest days and earliest memories. No one (not even lifelong partners) knows us in the same way. Since we know that as we age our long-term memory remains with us the longest, it is not surprising that older people retain those old images of themselves and their siblings.

Since I am next to the youngest in a family of five children, I have been surrounded by siblings for my entire life. It is hard for me to capture in words how much these relationships mean to me. I've also been thinking about how these relationships have aged. Over my lifetime, different siblings have played larger or smaller roles, depending partly on our geographic positions and partly on where we each were in our professional and personal lives.

When I was first married, my husband and I lived in the San Francisco area, not too far away from my older brother and his wife. As a result, my older brother was my first sibling to view me as an adult and peer instead of just a little sister. Along with sharing holidays with my brother and sister-in-law, my husband and I spent many a hilarious evening of drinking, attempting to play bridge, and talking about anything and everything. These evenings helped seal a bond of closeness for the four of us. I've always felt that their knowing my husband and me in the early days of our marriage has contributed to the connection we all still have to one another. We were young, and our marriage was new. They were family who loved and accepted us as we tried out our adult selves. We still laugh about the time I had way too much rum punch at their annual holiday party. I was a bit of an embarrassment to myself! But all those joint experiences and memories have helped build a strong bond that I treasure.

One of my sisters is four years older than I am. When I was born, the story goes that she wanted me for her birthday. (In fact, I arrived two days after her birthday.) Over time, we got used to sharing. We shared a room when we were young and shared clothes. Now we share thoughts and ambitions and ideas and whatever we feel like at the moment. Even though she still occasionally calls me "honey" (an endearing reminder that she's the big sister), our relationship is not about who's older or younger anymore. We both rely on the caring ear of the other and can count on open-minded listening when we need it. It's a relationship that has deepened and changed.

Grandparents/Grandchildren

Once I became a grandparent, I discovered a completely unique kind of relationship. Relating as a grandmother to our six-year-old granddaughter (and now beginning again with our new grandson) offers me the sheer joy of connecting to another person simply for the sake of the connection. I anticipate every interaction with my granddaughter with a kind of awe. What new thing will I learn from her young lips? What songs will I hear bubbling out of her? What will she teach me about her perspective on the world? There's a clarity and an openness when I interact with my granddaughter that require a specific kind of authenticity from both of us. I want to be precisely (or as close as I can get) who I am, and I want to accept her in exactly the same way. Being a grandparent teaches me daily how fresh, open, and free a relationship can be.

Another amazing part of being a grandma is the opportunity to see my son as a parent. I am moved by watching his patient, gentle, loving interactions with his children. I'll never tire of it. It warms my heart. And our daughter-in-law astounds us with how easily she trusts her precious children into our hands. What a gift she bestows with her relaxed acceptance of us and our grandparenting style.

Friendships Old and Young

After a wonderfully satisfying visit with a friend of over forty years, I got an e-mail from her that said, "One of the greatest joys of our senior years is the fellowship of long-held friendships and dear girlfriends."

I got to thinking about how important friendships have been to me over the course of my life. Writing about friendship should come easily for me, but I struggle to define the enormous values for me of having old friends. I couldn't live without these parallel relationships with people who are experiencing life alongside me.

Old friendships provide us a unique kind of sustenance. Unlike family relationships, they don't carry the baggage of genetic history, the intimate togetherness of families, or the fixed patterns of family behavior.

With old friends, we can let down our defenses. They have cheered our triumphs and been there for us when we have thrashed; they remember who we were when we were young and cherish us as we've changed and aged. Old friends know us in a special way unknown to others. Over time, I have learned that I can rely on them to understand me and my deepest thoughts and accept me—the bad and the good. Gaining this kind of trust takes years and years. Old friendships are one of the greatest perks of getting older.

Now that I'm in my sixties, I look back to the beginning of these longtime friendships. They began in so many different ways: as friends with babies the same age, professional contacts that developed into friendships after the work relationship had ended, neighborhood acquaintances that blossomed into close ties, school friendships, and powerful bonds formed when sharing a mutual loss such as the death of a loved one.

If I live to be very old, a consequence of forming these deep attachments will no doubt lead to heartbreaking pain when I face the loss of friends. Even though I realize the inevitability of such events, I find it hard to imagine life without these important relationships.

We never get too old to form new relationships. There's an old song: "Make new friends / But keep the old. / One is silver / And the other gold." While old friends may be the gold, new friends are also precious. Old friendships may be unique because of their longevity, but young friendships have their own special qualities. There is a freshness and a sense of adventure that come from discovering new alliances. Where will this relationship go? Will it last over time? We can relish that sense of potential.

I'm thinking of a "young" friendship that I have recently forged. I met Tracy through a professional connection. (This relationship is young in the sense that it is relatively new and in the fact that Tracy is considerably younger than I am.) At first we were meeting to give each other some peer supervision advice about our psychotherapy clients. We agreed that we'd meet monthly. This arrangement was hugely successful. Tracy is a talented therapist and could always give excellent insights into any of my cases. I was able to reciprocate with my interpretations of her clients' issues.

We quickly moved on from professional concerns to wonderful exchanges about our personal lives. We became friends. Tracy is one of the few people in my life who has actually pursued me. (I, so often, find myself in the pursuer role. It's a fact that I've spent many an hour in my own therapy, trying to analyze what this is all about.) In the case of Tracy, she would often assume the responsibility of making sure we got together regularly. It was important to her for us to have time together. It was a refreshing difference for me. I felt valued in a new way.

Now that years have passed since the beginning of our relationship, our friendship has blossomed, and we care deeply for each other's personal welfare. We've trusted each other with intimate family information and have stood by each other when either of us has found herself faltering or floundering emotionally.

Recently, Tracy faced a potential life-threatening diagnosis. As she was going through the tests to determine what she could expect, I got painfully in touch with how much her presence means to me. When she called to tell me that she, in fact, did not have a life-threatening disease, my relief was overwhelming. I learned a powerful lesson about how much I need this "young" friendship and all it offers me. How good to feel that I can continue to know and love this very special woman!

It seems a good idea not only to remain open to new or "young" relationships all our lives, but also to form friendships with people of differing ages. Having some friends who are younger than I is a way that I keep in touch with different segments of life and reminds me of issues that I have experienced in the past. These younger friends give me opportunities to behave as a wise elder. Some of my younger friends look to me as "the light at the end of the tunnel" as far as they peer at their prospects ten or fifteen years from now.

For me, seeing how a younger friend handles challenges that I too experienced broadens my vision of my own past. One of my younger friends has always seemed to be quite cognizant of her own needs while mothering several children. She expends tremendous energy in her job as mother but has found spaces and times to nourish herself with her friends and church group. When I was a young mother, I did not have this particular skill. The result was a feeling of being confined or trapped by my circumstances. These feelings led to a somewhat headlong rush toward the outside stimulation of work. Using my young friend's experience has helped me revise my own feelings of guilt or incompetence about that earlier time. I now see that it was natural to attend to my own needs and that there were all sorts of choices available to me to "feed" myself. Her younger perspective has taught me much.

Relationship building is an ongoing possibility for all of us. It need not be restricted by our physical health or mobility. We can continue to form and maintain relationships until the day we die. Even people with dementia can establish strong bonds with others. I've seen it in my practice—especially in my therapy through music. These connections with others can keep us stimulated, challenged, and truly engaged no matter how old we become.

CONTROL: ARE WE IN OR OUT?

For all of us, old or young, the issue of control over our lives is a daily challenge. Naturally, we attempt to exert as much control as possible. We need "to do" lists to help us make order out of chaos. We plan for the future. If we live to be old, we may find our options for staying in control of our lives increasingly limited. How do we prepare for this? Most of us would agree that it can be terribly anxiety-provoking.

Now that I am older, I wonder how much control have I had all along.

I have come to realize that there is (and always was) much that was outside of my control. There is the weather, for example . . . other people's driving, catastrophic illness, other people's behaviors, and on and on. While I've come to accept a lack of control in much that I encounter, I find myself feeling more and more strongly that the place to look for control in lives is within ourselves. We *are* able to have a say in how we behave and react. This quality seems to me to be the best path toward shaping the life we want and arriving at a place where we feel some control. This concept of responsibility for self permeates all areas of our lives: our work life, our relationships, our health, our inner peace. We want to feel we have some say in our own destiny. If we can begin to acknowledge this, it may lend us strength when we are faced with all those outside forces not in our control. Recognizing that we have chosen our own particular path can help us avoid blaming others (or the universe) for what we call our lives. It can help us see that we can be in charge of how we live. Claiming this kind of responsibility can be enormously freeing in old age. Believing that we control our own attitudes, we can sidestep regrets or wishful thinking about all the what-ifs of our past.

If we live to be old, we will need to address this issue of control. As our bodies age, we will likely lose some control over our physical beings. Our joints and limbs may not respond as they did when we were young. I recently fell while out walking and found it extremely disorienting and disturbing. It seemed so out of my control. (A ninety-eight-year-old woman in one of my music groups said, "Don't fall is our middle name!") Falling evokes fear and anxiety for anyone but particularly for the elderly. We can take precautions to avoid falling, and we may try to improve our balance. Taking an active stance is usually helpful. However, a misstep or trip can happen to anyone.

Falling is more than just an example of something that's out of our control. It may signify to an elderly person the impending ultimate loss of control: death. Certainly in the past, a fall often meant the beginning of the end—complications leading to death. While advances in the science of bone replacements and repair have zoomed ahead in recent years, the thought of falling may still haunt the minds of the very old.

How can the wisdom of aging help when contemplating or coping with loss of control? Acceptance of who we *are* and who we *are not* plays a big part here. With sixty-plus years under our belts, we can expect some perspective as we look back and view choices we have made. If we take time for introspection, we can begin to understand our own strengths and weaknesses and come to an acceptance of them. Using that knowledge of self, we can start assuming responsibility for our choices and make judgments about what really was or was not in our control.

Take, for instance, a choice of a life partner. If we made that choice as a young person, we did so with limited knowledge of what being together for an extended time entails. As we matured, we gradually discovered more and more about ourselves and about our partners. These discoveries might fuel an increasing stronger desire to remain with that person, or they might lead us to a conclusion that our own growth was being constrained by that person. We couldn't have known when we began the relationship. Only over time could the answers become apparent. How our partner changed and matured—though somewhat affected by us—would not be under our control. Only the passage of time would allow us the chance to separate what we controlled and what we did not.

As I have aged, I have found that many of the things I thought I controlled—like knowing how to choose the right partner to last a lifetime—were not actually in my control. What was in my control was my own responses to that person, my own behaviors in our interactions, my own attitudes toward what transpired between us.

As parents we attempt to control our children's upbringing. While we most certainly want to guide, care, and protect our children, another person (even a baby) is not really a person we can claim to control. Parenting provides countless opportunities to get a grip on what may or may not be in our control. From birth, a baby will have a part in determining his or her own future. Some babies (through body language) express a preference for cuddling and being held while others seem to need more distance from their parents and caretakers. From the beginning, these small people influence our interactions with them.

What experiences can each of us examine and dissect regarding control? Work situations might be a good possibility. While we can control our own efforts at competence, employee relations, work ethic, etc., we may not have control over who our superiors are, whether they possess good management skills, whether the company is moving in a direction that coincides with our own personal goals. Gaining an acceptance of what *is* or *is not* in our control will assist us in making choices about staying in a particular work environment or not.

My own work has offered me lots of opportunities to broaden my knowledge about what is or is not in my control. A while ago I got what I call a "kick in the head" lesson about control. A beloved client (whom I have known for over ten years) began to spiral down into a deep depression. Both her psychiatrist and I couldn't seem to find the right formula to interrupt the dramatic downturn. She was doing everything she could to help herself as she got sicker and sicker. We finally were able to get her admitted to a psychiatric unit, and over time, she was stabilized and has gradually returned to her higher-functioning self.

While I am thrilled that she has improved so much, I still remember the helplessness I felt as she became so ill. In the process of trying to help her, I allowed myself to become completely drained of energy. Looking back, I see that I struggled futilely to have some control over the situation—find some way to stop the chain of events. I wore myself out trying to achieve some kind of control over what was happening to another human being. What I've tried to accept in these days and months since is that no matter what my good intentions are, I need to be able to let go of the idea that I could somehow muster any control. One thing I know about myself is that I want to "rescue." This seemingly benign inclination can set one up to be conked on the head with reminders about control issues. My client offered me a powerful and painful lesson.

When interacting with others, it may be useful to acknowledge that the only real control we may have is over our own actions and behaviors. For each of us, how we have lived and the experiences we've had have shaped what those actions and behaviors may be. We may wish that another person would behave in a specific way, but we can't really control what that behavior might be.

Often when friends or clients tell me about painful interactions with spouses, in-laws, or others, I hear a yearning for the other party to change his or her behavior in some way. It's especially hard if we are standing by when a loved one is engaged in a self-destructive behavior. We feel our deep caring for the other person should be enough for them to change their ways. Don't they care enough about the relationship to make a change? In these cases, it seems prudent to remember that another person's behavior is really not in our control.

Still, it is possible to affect the outcome of an interaction by altering one's own behavior in the interaction. Particularly in long relationships, the two parties probably have developed over time a somewhat predictable behavior pattern with the roles becoming rather rigid. If one of the parties gradually begins to behave differently, the second party likely will attempt to maintain the status quo that has felt comfortable. However, if one-half of an interaction starts acting differently, the other half is nudged out of the old patterns, and a new dynamic can emerge.

Examining *fighting styles* for partners who have been together for a long time might be instructive. Most couples do engage in what some of us call "difficult discussions." It would seem almost superhuman for two people to live together for many years and *not* disagree. As time passes, couples' arguments often fall into a "fight pattern." This can be all right if both partners are able to emerge from the fight feeling relatively positive about the outcome, or that, at least, some bit of resolution has occurred. But if the aftermath of a fight leaves one of the parties feeling bruised and battered emotionally, then finding a way to change the pattern looms large. While we might wish for the other party to do the changing, the only person we really have any control over to do something is ourselves.

If, for example, one partner has a dramatic personality and the other half of the equation is a more subdued and introspective individual, it is very likely that their fighting styles might be very different. If our strategy for coping in an argument is to withdraw and pull back and our partner is more into getting anger out in the open with shouting and drama, then the likely outcome might be a stalemate. Withdrawing and becoming quiet may signal lack of engagement to the partner who may then rant and rave even more to get a response. If either partner can alter his or her behavior even slightly, it might allow for a different result. If the quiet one attempts to articulate his or her feelings and not shut down, or if the shouter chooses a quieter voice, a new pattern of fighting might emerge.

So often when people fight, they seem to lose their listening skills. I know that happens to me. Instead of trying to focus on what the other person is really saying, I'm busy attending to my own angry or hurt feelings. It may require outside help like therapy to help us get a grasp on our own actions and reactions. It's difficult to try to change an ingrained behavior pattern when we're not very sure what's driving it.

Efforts to feel in control can often lead to major disappointments and frustrations. We dwell on what we want or what we think is right, and then we're crushed when it turns out differently. I can look back to so many times that I presumed to know the feelings, attitudes, motives of someone else only to be knocked in the head by a totally different outcome. We are only one part of any interaction, and the possible actions and reactions of another are an unknown.

Expectations are tricky. If we had no expectations, we probably wouldn't accomplish very much. We expect ourselves to measure up. In fact, in my experience, most therapy clients come into therapy because their expectations of themselves or of others are not being met in some way.

Knowing ourselves well enough to avoid having unreasonable expectations can be liberating. It is also extremely easy to transfer our high expectations of ourselves onto those around us. Indeed, people with high self-expectations usually do have high expectations of others.

And having high expectations may set us up for disappointment, either in ourselves or someone else. I think part of what hit my mother so hard when my father died relatively young had to do with the fact that both of their mothers had died in their sixties and their fathers had lived much longer. In some way my mother expected the pattern to be repeated and that she would die before my father. When life handed her such a cruel reminder that we really can't know what to expect, she was especially vulnerable.

We can all think of times when we've eagerly anticipated some event or interaction with others only to be deeply disappointed with the actual outcome. We need to find ways to enjoy feelings of anticipation without being too specific or rigid about our expectations. This can be hard to do.

Like many of us, I look forward to family gatherings. Over time, I've tried to learn to let family events evolve into whatever shape they may take and to let go of specific expectations. I admit that I only accomplish this some of the time. Especially when it comes to our behavior within our family, we've had a lifetime to establish patterns and create our expectations of family members. Changing or easing up is not an easy task. Still, here is another place where our older age may assist us. We may be able to rely on our own raft of experience to adapt.

Sometimes I'm acutely aware that it's a good thing *not* to have control. When thinking about my adult children, I have my own opinions about what they should or should not do. I may question their actions. Eventually, I see their lives unfolding on their own timetables in their own unique ways, and I am relieved that their choices were not up to me.

Accepting a certain lack of control can be comforting. Most of the elderly people whom I have known work to preserve as much control in their lives as possible. Yet as their bodies and minds age, they are often called upon to give control over to others. It is how they accomplish this that interests me most.

How do the very old learn to relinquish control as they age? And how do they do it with grace? Thinking about and grappling with our attitudes toward control now can prepare us for the later time of old age. In my experience, the most contented older people have come to some kind of acceptance of what is and is not truly in their control.

Dependency Is Not a Bad Word

In the United States, much is made of the independent spirit. We learn practically from babyhood that it's good to be independent. We don't want to depend on others, and we want to feel we can do everything for ourselves. While I am a strong believer in taking responsibility for one's own actions, I have a different take on the word *dependency*. In most cases, we all probably live some sort of interdependent life. We rely on partners or friends for emotional support, for our social circle, and for our own definition of family. We *depend* on work colleagues for professional feedback and contributions to our career growth. We depend on others for all sorts of services in our daily lives. In my mind there is nothing all that wrong with the idea of dependency.

I can think back to many events in which some aspect of dependency played a part. Back in the 1970s, before I went back to school to get my social work degree, I worked as an executive director of an umbrella organization of women's rights groups. The president of the organization was a professional who volunteered her services. She was my boss and oversaw my work, which was carrying out the day-to-day business of the organization. This talented, generous woman taught me how to fulfill my duties. She was a patient editor, and I learned a great deal about writing from her careful attention to memos and letters that I wrote. Much of what I was required to do was new to me, and she guided me as I developed the needed skills. At the time, I was not aware of how much I depended on her; but looking back, I see how my dependence on her allowed me to gain confidence and skills that have served me ever since.

Still, the idea of being dependent when we are old can be distasteful. Over and over I hear people say, "I don't want to have to depend on my children," "I couldn't bear having to go to a nursing home," or "I hope I'll never need a wheelchair."

Being dependent need not have such a bad name. How often have we helped someone and felt that good feeling one gets from being helpful? Allowing others to do something for us is important. Some do it more gracefully than others. We can practice this art along the path to old age. Why wait until we're in dire need to allow someone to do a task for us that perhaps we could do for ourselves? Why not try dependency? Simple ways to try it out would be to say yes when a friend offers to help in some way, like offering a ride when your car is in the shop or offering a meal when you've been going through a stressful time.

While we are looking for ways to accept dependency, we may want to examine our own attitudes toward helping and being helped. What might it be that keeps us from letting others do things for us? Is it easy for us to allow someone to do something for us? Does it leave us with a feeling of obligation (a need to *pay something back*), or can we just accept it with grace? How do we feel about our own helpfulness? Do we like to be helpful or find it a burden? If we thrive on being helpful, can we accept help without needing to repay the help in some way? Do we need to help others as a way to feel OK about ourselves? What about gift-giving? Can we accept gifts from others easily? These and other questions may get us thinking about our ease, or lack of it, about dependency and give us clues to our own attitudes toward the idea of being dependent.

While each of us has our own personal response, some possibilities may include the following: (1) Allowing others to help us triggers a feeling of obligation; (2) Feeling dependent is linked with feeling helpless, powerless, or not in control; (3) Behaving dependently may be seen as weak.

Our bodies and minds change, and our abilities to perform tasks can change. Learning to accept the changes brought on by aging can be tough. The stories of my clients who gradually adapt to these changes have greatly broadened my own attitudes about dependency.

I have had the good fortune to witness many examples of how clients have dealt creatively with dependency issues. They have educated me in the various ways to effectively manage dependency and helped remove the possible stigma associated with being dependent. In particular, I am thinking of Claire, a woman I began to see for psychotherapy. She was in her midnineties when I started visiting her once a week.

Claire told me she was depressed. She seemed to have some good reasons for this feeling—she was blind and mostly bedridden. Her main diversion was listening to talking books, especially mysteries. Claire had lost her husband eight years prior to my meeting her and after a long marriage. Most of her friends were dead as well, and she had suffered the tragic loss of her beloved daughter in a car accident. She said she sometimes felt like the last leaf on the tree.

I had a resource book called *Writing Your Life*, which is a useful tool for life review. The book is a guide for helping people write their autobiographies and takes them through their lives chronologically, suggesting questions to get the person thinking. As I got to know Claire, we tried some of the suggestions. After a few sessions talking about her own life, Claire expressed an interest in doing some writing herself.

We then began a hugely satisfying period in our therapy work. She would dictate her thoughts, and I would write them down as well as I could. Then I would type them up and read them back to her at the next session. Over the week, between sessions, she would think about what would happen next in her story. She took some material from her life and wove it into fictional stories. She even tried her hand at writing a mystery.

I still have copies of Claire's finished stories, and when she died, I gave her writing to her family. While she needed to depend on another to be her eyes and transcriber, she chose an avenue of expression that afforded her tremendous satisfaction. She was a fine model for adaptability and an inspiration for me.

Another story of adaptability comes to mind: A friend, who has had numerous bone replacements, decided that maybe if she got a scooter, it would give her more mobility and freedom. It has, indeed, provided her more *independence*. Some might see her decision as giving in or becoming dependent on a machine for help. (One must keep walking, even if it becomes hazardous.) Now she is better able to go more places on her own and is less dependent on her partner for transportation.

Balancing choices to live life to the fullest is one of the big challenges we face as we age. When my mother chose to move to a retirement home at seventy-nine, she was extremely active and independent. She was still driving and led a busy life. As years passed, she aged in place and developed problems with her knees, which made walking more and more painful. She moved to the assisted-living section of her retirement home, but eventually, she just couldn't walk on her own. My family helped her make the decision to move into a facility with more care, and she graduated to a wheelchair. Of course being in a wheelchair limited her in many ways, but that wheelchair also gave her more mobility. We could take her out more easily. She no longer felt terrible pain moving from one place to another. Sometimes, what may seem at first to be a lessening of the quality of life (like needing a wheelchair) may evolve into something very different. Achieving some kind of balance allows us to stay engaged, calling upon the wisdom we've gained over the years.

A dear friend suffers from painful arthritis in her hands. She is very much an active, can-do person and a highly productive, resourceful woman. She is used to taking care of herself and others. I am impressed with how she has adjusted to having swollen fingers. She has shown a quiet acceptance of this consequence of aging and a willingness to ask for help when needed. She has always seemed to recognize the importance of attitude when dealing with health issues. While her attitude cannot change the fact of her arthritis, how she has adapted to it is a matter of mental outlook. By trying various strategies (some that have helped and others that have not), she has gained an acceptance of her condition. Digging down for the strength to accept what one cannot control can be key in tackling the challenges of an aging body. In a small way, she now may be more dependent or limited by what her fingers can no longer do. But what is significant is her adaptation technique.

A client of mine shows us how hard it can be to adapt to more dependency. This woman had been extremely independent. She raised her daughter and cared for her sick husband and ran a business with little outside help. Now in her 90s, she struggles daily with the difficulty of turning things over to her daughter and other facets that limit her independence. She has not had much experience learning how to depend on others, and at this period, it is difficult to learn. Because of failing eyesight and reduced mobility, she has no choice but to accept assistance. Even with little experience being dependent, she is marvelously resourceful and creative when coping with her diminishing strength. She makes an effort to learn caretakers' names in order to establish ties with them; she still tries to do as much for herself as she can manage, and she takes good care of her appearance in an effort to put her best face forward. Still, I wonder if sometimes asking for help over the course of her life might have prepared her more for the dependence she now feels.

Is it possible to experiment with dependency? I'm not sure. It might require too big a shift for some of us. We might have to consider outside help such as therapy.

I'm thinking of another client who, at seventy-nine, chose to try psychotherapy. She'd been her husband's caretaker during their long relationship. They had created a marital dynamic in which she was in charge of his chronic illness. She entered therapy at a time when she was realizing that her own health was now being affected by that lifelong pattern. She felt depressed when she viewed her future as more of the same. She began to examine herself and her own attitudes and tried to ease up on her expectations of herself. In therapy she articulated her feelings eloquently, almost poetically. One day she said to me, "Donna, I find myself looking up now when I go for my walks. I used to have my head down looking at my feet." What an astute metaphor for her gradual emergence out of depression! She literally felt things were looking up. In our time together, she began to look for ways to allow others to assume some of the burden of her caretaking role. This was not easy because even as a child, she had been expected to take responsibility for younger siblings in her family and had always been the dependable one. Shifting from being fiercely independent to depending, at times, on her adult children took effort. Trying to change such an ingrained behavior required a great deal of creativity and a strong desire for change. It was a joy to watch this client's movement toward a new kind of interacting.

My own mother was a fine example of gracious dependency. In the nursing home in the last year of her life, she adapted exceptionally well to depending on aides and nurses and family. She managed to get the care she needed without being too demanding and was genuinely appreciative when she received help.

Driving a car is an excellent example of how we maintain our independence. (Even the metaphor of propelling oneself forward speaks to the idea of independence.) I rely on being able to drive for all my professional work. Over and over with clients, I have witnessed the tremendous hardships of giving up driving. Often elderly people are not willing to quit, and family members and doctors must step in. Not driving limits one's independence drastically, so it is easy to see why an older person would resist this change.

However, a client of mine had the courage to decide on her own to give up driving. It took some struggling on her part to reach that conclusion, but her real motivation was not so much concern for her own safety but for that of others on the road. I admired her for making this tough decision. It has limited her options to some degree, but she has been exceptionally resourceful about getting around. She accepts offers of rides gracefully and then thinks of ways to pay the driver back, either with money or sometimes with an invitation to a meal. She has found drivers whom she can hire, and she has used public transportation more often. She acknowledges that it can be a terrific inconvenience, but her mostly cheerful acceptance has been a good model for me to remember if I may face this transition down the road.

Practicing the art of dependency when we're younger may ease the pain if we're faced with this major life decision. There is no need to wait until that time to accept rides. Rather than insist on independence when we're strong, we can choose to see what it feels like to let someone else drive us. Especially in the Washington area (but probably in most other places as well), there are numerous routes one can take to get from point A to point B. Everyone has a preferred route. If we're the passengers, it may take some self-control to sit quietly and let the driver navigate.

How do we practice dependency when we're actually fit and independent? There are lots of opportunities available. Sometimes just reframing an experience by thinking of it as dependency practice may help to take away some of the stigma about the word *dependency*. Little adjustments such as asking friends or adult children for help are good practices. Allowing a friend to bring dessert for a shared meal, accepting help with the dishes, accepting a ride instead of always being the driver are among the possibilities.

An old friend suffered a traumatic injury to his thumb while on a vacation. The accident meant that he needed to be evacuated from a river raft and taken for emergency treatment. Once home, he underwent a serious surgery to repair his thumb. After three weeks of healing time in a cast, he then began a painful round of physical therapy.

He was forced to depend heavily on his wife. Along with providing crucial emotional support, she had to drive him daily to the subway. The activities of daily living required that they each have enormous patience. He did make a full recovery. We have talked a lot about lessons that he and his wife learned. He discovered new degrees of patience and adaptability. As a couple, they found out how well they could manage a crisis together. Of course I'm not advocating intentionally injuring yourself. I'm only pointing out that there is always a wide variety of ways to view any experience.

I admit to sometimes choosing dependency. While I would readily sing the praises of computers (I got a Macintosh very early in the game), I have relied heavily on my husband's superior expertise and experience in using a computer. For me, a computer serves mostly as a glorified typewriter. As a result, my patience with glitches is next to minimal. While in the process of this writing, within a ten-minute time span, I both wanted help with the computer and insisted that I knew what I was doing. The outcome was (not surprisingly) humbling. I had misapplied our disc, which stored my documents, and I needed help unraveling my error. The whole experience got me thinking about how one can decide to accept another's help and then feel somehow incompetent or weak for *not* taking on the responsibility oneself. It's that complicated mix of dependence and interdependence that we all confront.

Perhaps it's all about balance—accepting help when we want or need it and balancing that with our need for independence. That sounds somewhat simplistic, but I imagine we struggle with that issue always, all the more so in our later years. It *is* possible to consider changing our attitudes about dependency *now*. Gaining some comfort with dependency early on might ease our way when dependency is no longer a choice. We may find that *dependency* is not such a bad word after all.

Illness as Opportunity

Is there a way we can look at illness as an opportunity? I think so. At the top of many people's lists of fears about their advancing age is the expectation of facing serious illness. As we age, we experience diminishing physical and mental power. At some point, our bodies and minds will begin to show signs of deterioration as do all living things. We will not live forever no matter what strategies we have for maintaining maximum physical fitness.

How can we find a new way to view illness or waning physical stamina? We may be able to see some of these struggles as opportunities. This attitude has made a huge difference to me as the years have gone by. It can bring new meaning to hard times.

Illness can actually be a unique opportunity for self-learning and a catalyst for change in our relationships with others. We may have to face the potential loss of a beloved family member and see that person in a new way. We may need to reevaluate our own bodies. We may find ourselves pushed to cooperate with other family members whether we want to or not; we may learn something wonderful about someone we've known all our lives. We may bond in totally unexpected ways.

A story about my husband and his brother is as follows: Sometime ago, my husband's brother was diagnosed with cancer. My brother-in-law was already ill at the time of his diagnosis, so it was a sort of double whammy for him. He lived alone in a tranquil seaside village in northern California and had retired from his longtime teaching position. However, he continued to write and give lectures on his passions: the environment and deep ecology. A well-known member of his community, he had a warm circle of supportive friends both from his academic life and his Buddhist temple.

My brother-in-law and my husband have lived very different, separate lives on opposite coasts. While their lives intersected during visits to their parents, they did not see each other with any regularity. After the deaths of both their parents, they made more of an effort to keep in contact. My brother-in-law became more and more committed to attending family events and flew back for a millennium Fourth of July gathering and attended my sixtieth birthday concert, even though his health was beginning to fail.

My husband is his brother's closest relative, and from the time he learned of his brother's cancer diagnosis, they remained in regular phone contact. Their connection began to strengthen as my brother-in-law's crisis became more and more apparent. My husband worked with his brother, a number of his loyal friends, the medical community, and social workers to construct a plan that would allow my brother-in-law to receive the necessary chemotherapy and radiation treatment he needed. My husband offered to be with his brother whenever he needed him, and my brother-in-law accepted the offer.

During those months when he was receiving treatment, my brother-in-law endured extreme nausea, fatigue, and excruciating pain from the radiation. He was terribly weak and frail, and we all feared we were losing him. My husband summoned all his creative caretaking talents to work for his brother during that terrible time. One of his saddest tasks was taking his brother's ailing twenty-year-old cat to be put down. They both loved that cat, and it had been a last living connection to their mother.

The intimate times that the two brothers shared during those harrowing months have allowed them to forge a lasting bond that did not exist before. Facing a life-threatening illness together granted them a special kind of closeness, which remains a facet of their current relationship. They shared an amazing victory of life over death.

What came into play here? Was it the fact that my brother-in-law allowed his brother to see him at his absolutely most vulnerable? Did it have to do with the trust established between them as my husband extended his help? What is it about feeling death lurking that prompts us to express ourselves in a different way? Does the finite nature of death lend an urgency to our interactions with loved ones? Do we fear time may be running out to express our feelings for one another? My brother-in-law's dire illness provided these brothers with a life-altering experience. The illness itself generated an intimacy that might not have occurred otherwise.

An eighty-year-old client, who has moved to the D.C. area to be near her three children, told a similar story about the impact of a health crisis on her and her family. When her husband fell and broke his hip and subsequently suffered a stroke while in the hospital, it quickly became apparent to her that she needed her children's help in coping with this crisis. (For years this woman had been very accustomed to being her husband's primary caretaker.)

With her husband's hospitalization, she got a glimpse of the strength and resilience of her adult children. They rallied around her and provided (thoughtfully and expertly) the support she needed. They became intimately involved in advocating for their father at the hospital and spent many hours with him. They exhibited loving sensitivity to her own needs for emotional and physical support by calling regularly and spending time with her as well. She seemed to recognize that a circumstance of this family health crisis was that she had precious one-on-one time with her children, which might not have happened in their regular day-to-day lives. She found a freedom to express to them some of her deepest feelings of pride and respect for them. She leaned on them and allowed herself to be bolstered by their advice and counsel. Her husband's illness served as the catalyst for an unusually intimate time for this family.

In a different context, a ninety-four-year-old woman told me that illness gave her an opportunity to learn how to rely on others. Now that she is very advanced in age, she is acutely aware of her physical limitations. She and her husband have a caretaker who comes in to help them seven days a week. This gentle man gracefully orchestrates their lives in most every detail. While the couple continues to do as much for themselves as they are able, they have gradually turned over more and more to this trusted employee. She seems to have achieved an easy acceptance of her own strengths and dependencies. Interestingly, when I asked her what she felt had helped her the most in dealing with her own aging, she immediately said, "Reading." She told me the world of books had transported her since childhood. She was an only child but never felt lonely. She pointed out that one is likely to spend much time alone if one lives to be old. Her childhood had prepared her for the aloneness of old age. For her, immersing herself in books is a vital occupation, one that greatly expands her now-limited horizons. Reading gives her opportunities to know other ways to live. All those stories of other people's lives help keep her mind open to new and different options.

Another story of illness precipitating a change in the dynamic between two people is a couple's description of how they managed when the wife suffered a debilitating fall. Before the fall, this couple was attempting to adapt to the husband's retirement, which meant he was at home much more, causing them to struggle with issues of space. She felt her house was being invaded, and friction developed as a result of their close quarters. After her injury, she required a good deal of care—especially as she worked to rehabilitate herself. As her husband took increasing care of her, they began to get more and more comfortable with their togetherness. She said that her illness afforded them an arena to find new ways to coexist.

Illness is very often labeled negative. These stories show us a different way to view it. Grappling with illness is not ever easy. Quite the opposite is true. But here again, our willingness to appreciate the lessons of illness can guide us.

For the very old, a specific illness may not be the issue so much as diminished strength and energy. I wonder sometimes why there is so much shame about the deterioration of our physical bodies. Is it really something we need to be ashamed of? Intellectually, we know that all living things will die, and unless they are cut down at a young age, all living things will deteriorate. So our options are either to die young and fit or to allow ourselves to deteriorate naturally. We can try to forestall deterioration, but our minds and bodies will lose strength as we age. What is so terribly wrong with that concept? Old trees must finally give way to this natural process. Our beloved old pets must be let go. Do we feel that humans should somehow be exempt from the fate of all living beings? Is it some kind of cultural abhorrence of what is aged or dying?

We as a culture tend to view aging as something to fix or cure, as if aging itself is a problem. Why is it surprising that people actually do become more frail late in life? We each have one lifetime.

An old friend had profound insights on what may be behind our shame about deterioration. "We are our bodies," she told me. "Our physical selves are at the heart of who we are." So as our bodies age (possibly becoming disfigured with painful arthritis, age spots, gimpy knees, etc.), we are constantly called upon to change our perception of self. We may look at our bodies in the mirror and not recognize that self we used to know. Our bodies will not allow us to ignore the passage of years and may scream at us to adjust our image of who we really are. Physical features (such as athletic limbs), which we have seen in ourselves as beautiful or strong, may change into parts of us that we now view with shame. Can we use the wisdom and experience of our older selves to transform these images of our aging bodies into beings deserving of acceptance, reverence, and love?

I talked with a woman about this, and she said she remembered photographing trees. The ones she found most interesting were the oldest ones—the ones with gnarled, twisted trunks. Is it possible for us to alter our view about this issue of human deterioration? Some kind of accommodation with it is crucial if we hope to reach a place of balance and equilibrium in old age. Personally, I lean toward seeing life as a circle. We are born and begin life as small beings who are weak and need care. We live and grow and become strong and mature. If we live to be old and die naturally, we no doubt will shrink and diminish, completing the circle.

A story about my daughter-in-law illustrates how an injury she suffered provided opportunities for us to deepen our bond with her. In what may turn out to be the worst summer of their lives, my son and daughter-in-law suffered multiple losses and anguish. Their beloved dog was diagnosed with cancer, and they knew they were going to lose him. His name was Trouble, and Trouble was no trouble to anyone. He was a loving, playful presence. He was a black Lab—a big dog who thought he was a lapdog!

In late May, my daughter-in-law came down the steps of her apartment building and, thinking she was on the last step, stepped down hard on her heel. She was, in fact, on the next-to-last step and, after a trip to the emergency room, found she had broken her heel. The treatment was three months of completely limited activity with her leg up. Within days Trouble began to fail, and they had to put him down. Our children suffered so from the loss of Trouble's wonderful presence in their lives.

Our children live in New York, and we're in D.C., so we tried to come up with ways to support them from afar. We committed to trying to call our daughter-in-law every day to check in on her and give her something to look forward to. These calls allowed us wonderful opportunities to get to know her. We could monitor how she was progressing and provide some outside stimulation for her. She looked forward to hearing from us, and we loved being "in" on our children's lives in a more day-to-day fashion. The usual circumstance (at least for us) is that our adult children's lives are so full with work and the business of life that we are not in such ongoing contact. That summer I went up to N.Y. twice to keep her company. These were special times where I felt useful, appreciated by both my son and his wife. My daughter-in-law's painful injury had side benefits that none of us would have predicted. One benefit was that it taught them how to manage as a couple with a serious health issue. My son turns out to be a skilled, creative caretaker, and my daughter-in-law is a very plucky, feisty patient. Our children have now had some practice with how they handle a serious health condition.

How we have dealt with our own health issues may give us an idea of what our approach may be in later life. What kind of patient have we been? How do we handle pain? Can we accept caretaking or ask for help when we feel ill? Do we have any experience being sick? Do we take our own health for granted? Answering questions like these may give us a clue as to how we might manage failing health in old age. We might even be able to see our own or another's illness as an opportunity.

Grief and Loss

Every change always has a component of loss. Even happy changes, such as the birth of a baby, involve both gain and loss. Think of the advent of a child into a family and the changes it produces. One of the first losses it creates is a big loss of sleep! But when we look deeper, we recognize other losses—like the transformation the new parents go through from being a couple to becoming a family. Their lives are altered forever. The couple loses the time they used to have as a twosome. They take on new roles that may feel awkward at first. Even the loss of space in their living arrangements is a change.

Changes force us to deal with loss all through our lives, and that may help us cope with the losses of aging. If we can examine our own style of dealing with loss, it can help us when losses begin to pile up. It is likely that we will cope with loss and grief in our own particular way. If our usual mode is to talk things over with people, express ourselves outwardly, and seek help in times of crises, then it's likely we will turn to these strategies when faced with a huge loss. If we tend to need activity to keep us grounded, we will find ways to be active. If we usually cope by mulling things over privately, we will probably be more private with our grief.

I have been greatly impressed by elderly clients who have suffered numerous losses and seem to have the ability to plow through their grief to a place where they can rejoin others. In my work as a social worker with the elderly, I have been privy to all sorts of effective (or sometimes ineffective) approaches to dealing with loss.

For a woman whom I met when she was in her seventies, the long-ago loss of her mother was still so acute she cried a lot. The nursing home approached me about working with her, using music as a therapeutic tool. She had been a civilian worker for the military in Vienna after World War II.

She loved opera and Viennese waltzes. We decided to listen to opera (her favorite was Rigoletto) and Strauss waltzes. Using the music to open her up, we began to talk about her life and her memories of her mother. Hearing opera in her home as a child was one way she deeply connected with her mother. Over time, she cried less and less and appeared more at peace with the death of her mother. Her experience with the music reminded me of a passage from Ethan Canin's novel *Carry Me Across the Water*: "Music transported him. That was the word. It brought him straight to his loss. Somehow, this was a comfort."

Music reached this woman in a powerful nonverbal way that allowed her to release her long pent-up grief. She was able to capitalize on her own love of music to achieve a positive change.

Another woman who always participated in my music groups at her assisted-living facility was nearing ninety when she lost her beloved daughter to cancer. She clearly felt the loss strongly and spoke with sorrow about her loss. Over time, she was able to recover and carry on. She was a beloved resident and thrived on her connection with the staff and the other residents. Her usual style of staying engaged with others helped her move through her loss.

While it sometimes may appear that the very old don't show the pain of their losses in the same way that we who are younger do, it's my opinion that their age has allowed them to develop quiet ways to cope and altered their perspectives about their losses. If we are faced with accumulating losses, it seems to me we would eventually "lose" ourselves if we allow loss to swamp us. Older people have achieved some kind of accommodation with grief and loss and its natural place in their lives. They seem to expect it and, therefore, accept it more readily.

For me, one of the most salient features of loss is its unpredictability. While we can speculate on what a loss might be like, it is not really possible to know until we actually experience it. Accepting this fact of unpredictability could encourage us to let go of some of our fears about grief. If we can't know now what it will be like, we might as well wait till it's a reality and deal with it then. Even losses that are expected, like the loss of an aged parent, can take us by surprise. When my mother died at the age of almost ninety-one, we all were expecting to lose her. She had gradually declined and literally sort of faded away. She was in a coma for the last weeks of her life, and hospice had told us what to expect at the end. After she died, I assumed that I would be greatly comforted by my memories of her. What was so surprising was that immediately after her death, I really didn't want to remember because every memory was a painful reminder that she was gone. Now, after many years have passed, I welcome every incident that reminds me of her.

The unpredictability of grief seems to me to be inevitably tied to the unpredictability of death and may be, in an odd way, a kind of rehearsal for the ultimate loss we'll face: our own death. As we live, we have gained tremendous experience dealing with all kinds of losses. We each can point to any number of losses that we have already experienced: from the deepest pain of losing a precious loved one to the more mundane frustration of losing our keys. If we choose to look at all the losses in our life as practice, we can begin to gain some confidence that we *do* know something about it.

My husband (of forty-five years) and I discuss what it might be like to be widowed. While I can try to imagine a life that would not include him, I have no idea what my universe would be like without him. So much of my life would change. I would have to adjust to a markedly new world and adapt to a new *me*. It sounds exhausting and unbelievably painful. Loss and grief *are* exhausting.

Over and over, clients, family, and friends mention the tremendous fatigue and disorientation of grief.

What we *should* be can be a huge stumbling block when we're grieving. People who have suffered a major loss need to work through their grief in their own time span. It's very difficult to measure that from the outside. Religions offer timely rituals that may help, but in the end, it is still an individual process. We, who are on the outside, see the grieving person through our own eyes and experience. It's impossible for us to know another's experience. We can empathize and listen, but refraining from judgment may be the best gift we can offer the grief-stricken.

The losses of aging, of course, go beyond losses of loved ones. In conversations I've had with friends and family, they tell me the loss of physical vitality, mobility, and other health issues top the list of concerns. As our bodies change, we grow more conscious of the aging appearance. While we continue to do the best we can with our outside image, we may need to adapt to a more mature view of what is attractive.

One friend talked about his aging appearance and "old knees." He clearly did not like the way aging was changing his body. Feeling good about our changing bodies is tough. We remember what we used to do with ease and mourn the loss of physical agility. The longer we live, the more wear and tear we must suffer. As our minds mature and gain wisdom, our bodies, in contrast, will be deteriorating. Perhaps we can look at our increasing wisdom, knowledge, and expertise as a way of balancing against our diminishing physical prowess.

What is it that will grant us the ability to view ourselves and the changes in our bodies with more compassion? How can we ease up on our expectations of ourselves to continue functioning as we did twenty years ago? What can lead us to an acceptance of, and appreciation for, our *selves* no matter how old we become?

One answer might be to see our bodies as teachers. We need to trust what our bodies can tell us about ourselves. This physical aspect of our *selves* has stored fantastic information about us since the day we were born. All of us may have experienced the consequences of not listening to our bodies. They often literally cry out in pain, asking us to change our ways.

When I was younger, I suffered from terrible migraines. They always forced me to suspend whatever I was trying to do that day and seek a dark, quiet place to recover. The relief I experienced when the migraines were finally over was exquisite. Now, even though I can control these headaches with miracle medicine, I look back and speculate that those migraines provided me solitary peace and quiet, which I needed at that time in my life. (I still need that kind of time for myself, but I've found healthier ways to achieve it.)

Our bodies have so many messages for us if we stop and listen. As in the case of my migraines, each of us can find ways to pay attention to bodily advice. Fatigue may be a sign that we must alter the use of our time and find ways to allow more rest. Recurrent symptoms also may have hidden meanings if we take a look.

If we think about it, we know our bodies better than anyone else. Even trusted medical personnel cannot fully know what it's like to live in our skin. My mother-in-law was a good teacher on this concept. She knew she was extremely sensitive to medications. When her doctor prescribed something new, she always monitored herself for possible side effects. In this way, she utilized her trust in her own knowledge of her body as an advocate for her own health.

Since aging means dealing with *transitions*, we need to remember that transitions always carry with them a by-product of loss. At least in my case, I am more and more aware every day of the element of change. My granddaughter seems to change every time I see her. My own body develops a new ache here and there. Relationships are in a constant state of flux. It's hard to follow all the changes happening in my friends' lives. While change can have the excitement of something new, it can be hard to face the accompanying feelings of loss of the old.

Recently, friends sold the house they'd lived in for years and moved to a beautiful waterfront area where they had built a new home. Their move caused me and many of their friends to look hard at what it's like to pack up years of living in one place and completely alter how one lives. In many ways, they have been trailblazers for those close friends around them. The grief associated with major life changes, such as selling the house one has lived in for thirty-plus years, may be acute.

Not many weeks after this major life transition, my friend's mother died at age ninety-six. My friend commented that her mother's death so superseded her other losses that it somehow helped her move on through them more easily. Who could know in advance that the timing of her mother's death would grant her such a perspective?

The whole process of sifting through one's accumulated belongings may actually aid in the gradual acceptance of this change. Periodic cleanouts of possessions might be a good idea for developing some familiarity with the task of disposing of material things and sorting through the complex emotional ties to those things. For me, the need for, and attachment to, material things has decreased as I've aged. I have noticed a desire to "lighten up."

An eighty-year-old client gave me a gentle lesson in the concept of lightening up. I had given him a vase of roses for his eightieth birthday. The next time we met, he came out to the car with the vase in his hands. When I told him the vase was part of the birthday gift, he said he really didn't need any more "things." I got his point.

It may be that as we age, we will begin to want to shed some of the material things that we have collected over our lives. It may be part of a kind of paring-down process leading ultimately to the simplicity of death. When we're young, we are far more desirous of acquiring and adding to our lives. We want to acquire our own house with appropriate furnishings. We may want to add to our family. We acquire experiences. Later we can look at what we've amassed. We may begin that process of paring down, simplifying, the lightening up my client taught me about.

A small example of this concept was a funny experience we had when we redid our twenty-year-old kitchen. While the work was in progress, we camped out, using a small kitchen in our basement. We made do with a few plates, minimal cooking equipment, and much-simpler meals. When our beautiful new kitchen was finished, we were struck by how well we had managed with so little! Did we really need all that space after all?

Bringing grief to conscious awareness may be needed to help us deal with it. My dad died when he was fifty-seven and I was twenty-three. At twenty-three, I didn't know much about coping with such a loss. After the funeral, I went on with my life. For years I found myself crying in the summers (he had died on June 26) with no awareness of why that was happening. Twenty years later, I became involved with a center whose focus was helping people with grief, loss, and dying. With some counseling at that time, I connected my tears to the long-ago loss of my dad. By bringing my grief to the surface, I was more able to work through it. Recognizing a need to cry as an avenue of release is one way to access what our real feelings are. Then allowing ourselves to have a good cry could be a next step. The concept of being comfortable with crying (either one's own tears or another's) has a long way to go in this society. We all are probably fairly expert at repressing feelings, especially sadness. We may view crying as a sign of weakness. However, tears are a natural way to let down and let go. I've given some thought to the question of which people in my life seem comfortable with my tears. It's a real gift when a person can stand by and keep emotionally separate enough to let me weep.

An article in the *New York Times* Arts section (August 27, 2006) about John Kander and Fred Ebb (a songwriting duo for forty-two years) contains beautifully articulated advice about facing the losses of aging. Kander and Ebb wrote many famous musicals including *Chicago, Cabaret,* and the *Kiss of the Spider Woman*. The article discussed the complexities of their professional relationship and focused on a new production called *Curtains,* which later came out in Los

Angeles. During their work on *Curtains*, Ebb died. Kander (who is seventy-nine) spoke about this huge loss and how he finally was able to return to work without his lifetime collaborator. "I made this switch in my head, quite consciously. Instead of dealing with it as a big trauma and a big cry of grief, I started to think of it as just a different chapter. You have to get used to losing things in life, or you're done for."

The writer of the article went on to describe Kander remembering what, at first, seemed like his unrelated childhood memories. He remembered the time his aunt Rheta put her hand over his to teach him his first chord: C major, and the season, even earlier, that he spent isolated on a sleeping porch, recovering from tuberculosis. "I've always thought that I became a listening person then," Kander said, "listening for the sounds of footsteps coming toward me."

As this *New York Times* writer put it so eloquently, "If your ear was tuned to the frequency of human contact, it was necessarily tuned to the frequency of human absence as well. Love and loss were not separate channels."

"Once I acknowledged that," Kander said, "I felt free to go to work."

My work has afforded me excellent opportunities to experience what grief and loss look like. That in itself has been a kind of preparation for my own future losses. By choosing to work with people nearing the end of their lives, I selected a career that would require me to learn how to say good-bye. It was an unconscious choice at the beginning, but now I recognize the huge value it has provided for me. Often my relationships with clients have lasted over a period of years, and my attachments to them have been deep. The difficult process of letting go of these relationships has become somewhat familiar. That fact lessens my terror and fear of loss to a degree. It gives me some experience with what a final parting with someone I care about might feel like.

I had some painful practice of this sort when I had to say good-bye to Mr. James. I knew Mr. James for almost twenty years. He and I never could seem to remember accurately the exact beginning of our relationship, but we both knew it covered a long time. When I met him, he was in his sixties (a time of life that is now my own). Through my care management work with him over many years, we developed a close, deeply connected relationship. In the beginning, I was very involved with his care, but gradually his guardian took over those duties, and I became more of a source for social interaction and outside stimulation for him. His memory about the history of Washington, D.C., was stunning, and I gleaned wonderful stories about the old days in the city. Much of our time together was spent on outings to various gardens, historic monuments, or cultural events in the Washington area. We shared a mutual interest in so many things. Our rapport became finely tuned, and we both looked forward to our meetings.

Now Mr. James has passed his eighty-second birthday. As he has aged over these twenty years, so has his guardian, who has now retired and has moved away from the D.C. area. Mr. James moved with him. So I had to say good-bye to this man with whom I had become so deeply attached. We had always celebrated his birthday together, so I planned a birthday lunch. My heart was heavy as I drove to pick him up for what would be our last outing. It was hard to feel celebratory. We enjoyed our lunch in one of his favorite restaurants, but I found myself thinking back through the years and noticing how much he had aged. Just getting in and out of the car was now so much more of an effort than it was for the man I had known twenty years ago. (He had developed Parkinson's disease over the years.) His sharpness had faded.

We took one last drive around some of the sights in D.C. All the time I kept thinking, *This is the last time we'll do this together*. I tried to keep my tears at bay. In our time together, we talked about how long we'd known each other and remembered some of those moments. When we got back to his apartment building, we got out of the car and walked slowly up to his apartment door. As we walked down the hall to his apartment, I tried to match my steps to his painfully slow gait. We went into his apartment. I gave him a picture of us taken many years ago when we had gone to see the FDR Memorial when it was new. (I have this same picture in my office.) We hugged, and it was impossible not to shed some tears. I waited while he slowly lowered himself into his chair, and then we said good-bye. I cried the whole way back to my car, and I still mourn the loss of this dear man.

While I doubt that I will see Mr. James again, I have no doubt that he will remain with me in my memory and in my heart. Each encounter with another person leaves its mark upon us. We retain the traces of these interactions forever—sometimes consciously, and sometimes not. Still, I find this thought has been a huge comfort for me as I've had to let go of clients who have left or died.

While grief and loss are integral parts of all of life, they magnify as we age. Trusting our own experience with grief and loss over time can shore us up as losses accumulate.

On Dying and Death

Whatever course our life has taken, the reality is that our journey will ultimately come to an end. It's entirely feasible to not contemplate one's death, but the fact is that we will go ahead and die whether we choose to contemplate it or not. But I have found that those who have gained some acceptance of the finiteness of life are also those who most recognize its preciousness and make the most of the time that they have.

As my friend Jack said, "Everybody dies." The inevitability of death is not exactly startling news. Yet I encounter those who feel they may be somehow exempt from this universal end. While musing on death may be scary, it needs to be part of our mental process as we move toward old age.

Awareness that our lives will ultimately end helps us define who we are in the time between now and that end. Keeping in mind that we have limited time on this earth can serve as a prod to make the most of life. Each of us has only this one chance (except for those who believe in reincarnation) to assemble a life.

Becoming older (and therefore closer to my own death) affects my choices about how I spend my time. Reminded that my time is finite, I am less likely to choose to spend it with people who sap my energy or exude negativism. Less and less do I choose to engage in activities that I do not value. Fewer things are "shoulds," and many more choices are conscious.

Looking at the losses of loved ones, we can see how this concept of the finality of death can come into play. Death helps to crystallize our picture of those people. When someone's life ends, everything from then on is defined differently in our minds. We must adapt to a new world with an empty space. Death is a very specific demarcation. It alters our perception of time. We begin to think in terms of "before the person died" or after the death.

Finiteness can be clarifying, as George Will wrote in a moving column about the death of his mother (*Washington Post*, July 13, 2006), who died at the age of ninety-eight after "her body was exhausted by disease and strokes. Dementia, that stealthy thief of identity, had bleached her vibrant self almost to indistinctness, like a photograph long exposed to sunlight."

Not too long ago, my husband accompanied his brother who was moving toward the end of his life. It was an amazing odyssey requiring tremendous strength, trust, and sacrifice for both brothers. After his brother died, my husband experienced over and over that clarity that George Will mentions. His picture of his brother has been continually redefined as he hears new stories and anecdotes about his brother. He expects to broaden his view of his brother's life until he comes to his own death.

If we choose to ponder death, experiencing our own death is the ultimate relinquishing of control (if we set aside the choice of suicide). This experience of gradually letting go of various aspects of our lives may be precisely the preparation we need for the final letting go of death.

How one goes about dying seems to loom much larger for many than the fact of death itself. They worry about the form their dying may take. Those who have watched an aged parent linger on and on through an excruciatingly slow demise have experienced firsthand how hard that particular kind of dying (or should we say living?) can be. One friend spoke of how her mother had "outlived herself."

One way to try thinking about death is to gain some comfort with the huge range of possibilities for ways to die. This knowledge may relieve some of our anxiety about what our own departure from this world might be like. Witnessing the deaths of many elderly clients has given me familiarity with death in its different forms. Knowing more about an unknown (and in this case, the ultimate unknown) can lessen our fear. Because my work demands that I interact with the dying and those around them, I have been granted an opportunity to see what different kinds of dying (or living till one dies) may look like. This witnessing has made the subject of death less threatening, less off-limits, more familiar, and more acceptable for me.

We all aspire to a "good" death (along with a good life) for ourselves and for loved ones. In my experience, the definition of a good death can be all over the map. There are as many kinds of deaths as there are births. Just as a birth is uniquely individual, so is a death.

I am reminded of a client I saw quite a long time ago who was Czech and had limited English. He suffered from Alzheimer's and would become agitated and difficult for the staff to deal with. He had been a trained singer in his past. The nursing home hired me to work with him, using music in the hope that it might help calm him. I thought he might want to sing with my accompaniment. But as is the case with many singers, he wasn't happy with his aging voice. Instead of encouraging his singing, I began to bring in CDs of Schubert songs for us to listen to together. He was far more familiar with this genre than I was. The work evolved into a lovely relationship in which he taught me much about Schubert song cycles and vocal music in general. He understood all the German language in the songs, so his lack of English was not important. We communicated through the music.

As we worked together, we developed a pattern for our sessions. We always listened to Schubert's "An die Musik" at the beginning of our time together. This exquisitely lovely song ("To Music" is the translation of the title) speaks of the amazing power of music. The words are as follows:

Thou lovely Art, how often in dark hours,
When life's tumult wraps me round,
Have you kindled my heart to loving warmth
And transported me to a better world!

Often a sigh, escaping from your harp
A chord, sweet and holy from you,
Has opened up a paradise for me,
Thou lovely Art, I thank thee for this gift!

After many months of only listening to the CDs, I brought in Schubert's "Ave Maria" and tried playing the piano part to see if he might try singing it. He began singing just the words *Ave Maria* (which are actually a lot in that particular piece). Although he might have felt his voice was not up to his standards, it really was quite a lovely baritone voice. One day when he was singing "Ave Maria," I looked up to see a staff person standing and listening. She had tears running down her cheeks. He had touched her with his music.

For this particular man, the music was a pathway to his heart. If he was agitated when we began a session, he would become noticeably calmer during our time together, and the staff remarked on the change in him when he would return to his unit. I knew him over the course of about two years. When he began to deteriorate physically, the staff informed me that they felt the end was near. I went to see him at the nursing home. He was in bed, and he was not responsive. I decided to play recordings of "An die Musik" and "Ave Maria" for him and sat quietly with him, holding his hand, as the music washed over us. The words of "An die Musik" seemed so poignant and relevant. He died the next day. In my mind, his was a "good" death.

Twenty-some years ago, I received training from the then St. Francis Center (now called the Wendt Center) to become what was called a "caring volunteer." It was an intense weeklong training covering many aspects of death and dying with the purpose of preparing me to become a companion for someone with a terminal condition. We participated in such exercises as writing our own obituaries and a guided imagery in which we imagined our own dying and contemplated the idea of choosing who we'd have with us if we were dying. We were educated by people who had survived cancer and who had lost a child and others with personal experiences relating to the process of dying. I credit that long-ago training for equipping me to work with the very old. The topic of death and dying went from being an unknown to a known. The more I've experienced the repeated losses of elderly clients, the more I've learned about the different styles that people use to leave this world.

People often asked me if it was depressing to work as a caring volunteer or to work as a social worker with the very old. For me, the opposite is true. When working with someone in the last part of his or her life (whatever the age), you have the priceless opportunity to be in touch with *life* at its most intense. It's the "living" of the dying person that can teach us so much. Those who know that their deaths are approaching seem to live as close to their core selves as is possible. They have set their priorities and attempted to tie up the loose threads of their lives. Often the dying seek opportunities to mend broken relationships or forgive old wounds. If we have access to them in their last days and hours, we are privileged. We may, through observation, learn much from the dying about how to live.

My husband had the painful but moving experience of losing a dear friend after a long battle with cancer. In his last months, his friend welcomed weekly visits from my husband and another man to whom he was also close. Over the weeks that these three men spent together talking, laughing, and sometimes crying, my husband participated in the profound process of watching how a loved person lived till he died. His friend graciously shared the extremely private act of his dying. For my husband, that felt like a gift, and he savored those last conversations and moments. Time in his friend's bedroom was a kind of "time out of time." Those meetings were separate from the daily rush and activity of life and carried the unspoken knowledge that they would end with death. The shared intimacy was unlike anything my husband had experienced previously. In a way, it was a form of "death education," which is now a part of my husband's memory and thinking. His friend served as a model for him.

My husband's friend was comfortable talking about his impending death. He had deep religious beliefs, which added to his comfort with the topic. How to broach the subject with a loved one who is dying is a common dilemma for family and friends. While it seems it might be beneficial for both parties to have a chance to talk about the dying, most often we need to take our lead from the person who is facing death. It is after all *his or her* death, not *ours*. The dying person deserves to choose his own way of dying. This applies as well to the issue of saying good-bye. There is much written about saying our final good-byes. Again, we are confronted with whether our loved one offers opportunities for these farewells. While we do not want to impose our own needs on the dying, we may discover other ways to say good-bye, such as a written message expressing our feelings.

I remember the months leading up to my father-in-law's death. He had suffered a series of strokes, which affected his memory and caused him to be disoriented at times. At the time that he was failing, I was working with a therapist, and he strongly advised me to go to my father-in-law to tell him good-bye. (I had never been able to say good-bye to my own father because he had died suddenly many years before.) I flew out to California for a last visit with my father-in-law. I can remember feeling extremely anxious about how I could begin a conversation that would lead to my saying good-bye to him. In the end, he made it easy for me and created an opening that allowed me to speak up. I can't recall the specific words I used, but I vividly remember looking into his eyes and sensing his love and understanding. He seemed to comprehend that we would never see each other again.

My father-in-law was in a coma for several weeks before he died. It was a painful time of waiting for all of us, especially my mother-in-law. What I found extraordinary was what my mother-in-law told me about his dying. She had spent so many hours at the hospital with him as he lay comatose. The day before he died, she said to him, "This is no way for you to live." He died the next day. She felt, in retrospect, that she had been holding on to him, and he had stayed with her until she could release him from this life.

The first client I had who died was a plucky ninety-year-old lady. I had done a lot of practical care-management kinds of things for her—helping her grocery shop, taking her to doctor's appointments, etc. We had developed an easy, comfortable relationship. She was quite straightforward and direct about her needs, which made it easy to assist her. She discovered a lump on her neck, and when they did a biopsy of the mass, they found it was malignant. At age eighty-nine, she elected to have radiation treatment, and I drove her to most of the treatments. (It was a big education in what radiation does to human skin.) The treatments did not halt the progress of the cancer, and she moved from her apartment into a nursing home. In my last few visits with her, she was quite matter-of-fact about her impending death. She was very comfortable talking about it. That fact helped me open the topic, and it allowed us to establish a special kind of intimacy. It was acknowledged between us that she was "leaving." The finiteness of our time together seemed to break down some of the barriers that can exist between people. We both knew our time together was limited in the most powerful way. The last time I saw her was the day before I was leaving on a trip. (So in an odd way, I was the one who left.) It was our best visit since she had moved to the nursing home. She was awake and alert. I got to tell her that I loved her and gave her a little finger wave as I left her room. She finger-waved back. I sensed that it was unlikely I'd ever see her again. While I was away on my trip, I got the message that she had died. How lucky I was to have such a wise teacher about the art of dying.

Washington Post humorist Art Buchwald had a remarkable experience with dying and living to tell the tale. When his doctors said his kidneys were failing, he elected not to go on dialysis and entered a hospice for his last days. Well, his days lasted into weeks and then months. He continued to write some columns while he waited for his death. In one hilarious example (*Washington Post*, April 6, 2006) called "One Glorious Sunset," he talked about becoming a celebrity, "the only person who got famous for dying." He was interviewed by Diane Rehm. George Stephanopoulos had Buchwald on his show, and then Sharon Waxman wrote a long piece about him in the Sunday *New York Times*. (As Buchwald points out, "You never existed unless you get into the New York Times.") Buchwald acknowledged that "when you are in a hospice, people are very curious about you, about themselves and about how to deal with denial."

His experience again shows how a dying person can act as a catalyst and inspiration for people to ask questions and open the topic of death to discussion. Surprisingly, Mr. Buchwald improved enough to leave the hospice, return to regular writing for the *Post*, and complete a book about his experience. He said his mantra was, "I've put death on hold."

For me, thinking about death has increased as I've aged and moved nearer to it. These thoughts help remind me daily of my life. The idea of my own end pushes me to live as fully as possible *now*; to use my remaining time with conscious choices about time; to try to appreciate breathing, walking, seeing, hearing, loving—all those aspects of being alive that we can so easily take for granted.

Yin and Yang

Let's consider one last notion in our quest for the fullest possible older age. It's the idea of yin and yang—borrowed from Eastern philosophy. The Chinese characters yin and yang literally mean "the shady and sunny side of the mountain." I've always thought of it as the dark and the light, the cool and the warm. The whole of everything is comprised of opposites, or more accurately, what is shady on the mountain gradually turns to feel the sun as the earth rotates on its axis. It can be enormously freeing to consider that everything we experience can be seen to contain both the light and the dark.

This can allow us an ever-expanding view of our lives. I have found that when I am hurt or angry during a personal interaction, it can be extremely useful to try to see the situation from the opposite perspective. What is going on for the other person? What prompts another's behavior? What, other than my hurt, is going on here? Taking this tack invariably gives me some distance and new insights about what may be transpiring between us. This perspective can work in any occasion that feels difficult, painful, or stuck.

We can apply this idea of yin and yang in an infinite number of ways. It can allow us to see positives in negatives and "goods" in "bads." For instance, when I used to think about stubbornness, my first instincts were to think difficult or mulish. But Martha, a therapist, gave me a new way to look at it. Martha spoke approvingly of her aging mother who had a lifelong pattern of being stubborn. Although her mother's stubbornness certainly could be difficult to deal with, in Martha's enlightened perception, she also saw the other side of her mother's stubbornness. It seemed to be a way her mother was able to preserve her identity as she became weakened by advancing age. Her mother's obstinacy forced aides and others around her to see her as a separate individual and not just as a "case." Her mother's stubbornness helped her hold on to her persona. Rather than just the "woman in room number 26," Martha's mother showed personality, a uniqueness that distinguished her from other patients. While aides might have labeled Martha's mother as stubborn with a negative connotation, the stubbornness itself became a useful quality of differentiation.

Let's look at anger with this two-sided perspective with no label of "good" or "bad." Coping with anger is a task with which we can all identify. It can be scary, whether it's our own anger or someone else's. There's always the chance of its getting out of control. Still, anger can be a motivating force and may be just the emotion we need to nudge us into positive changes.

Feeling growing anger and frustration at work might be just the internal push we need to activate us toward new employment. That seemed to work for one of my sons. He had high hopes as he started out with a young company. He liked his work and grew in the job until he felt extremely confident and competent doing the work. Over time, though, his hopes of advancement were not realized. The company's management never really carried through on the plans they had once held for the company's expansion. Good managers left the company. My son became more and more dissatisfied and frustrated, and those feelings grew into anger. When he realized he was angry, he was also able to look at the other side, the *cause* of his anger, and could see for the first time that it was time for him to find a new situation.

The expression of anger within a family can also lead to a rearrangement of family relationships, if we can see both sides of what the anger is really all about. My younger brother and I are two years apart and really grew up linked together while our three older siblings were thought of as a somewhat separate unit. (Family vacations either involved the three older brothers and sisters or us.) In our adult lives, my brother and I had increasingly less-regular contact, and I missed our old closeness and connection. Then an incident occurred that made me quite angry with my brother, and it turned into a painful scene. Over the next few months, we had some honest phone conversations in which I was able to express why I was angry, and he stayed open to listen and respond. Ultimately, I was also able to express my feelings of loss about our lack of contact. We struggled through a tough time, but my initial expression of anger had opened the door to clearing the air and renewing our bond.

Let's consider other attributes that we may tend to label as either just positive or just negative. Stoicism is usually thought of as a good quality. We admire people who are stoic and endure pain without a lot of complaining. No one loves a whiner. And there is the idea that living through pain can make you strong. On the other hand, pain may be a valuable signal from our bodies or our minds. Pain may have a message for us that we need to make some sort of change or attend to ourselves in some way.

I am friends with a lovely young woman who didn't notice both sides of her own stoicism and suffered unnecessarily because of it. Deborah is a person who performs pretty much 100 percent in whatever she chooses to do. She gives 100 percent to her role in her family and 100 percent to her demanding job. It's not surprising that all too many 100 percents add up to tremendous stress on her, mentally and physically. She recently gave in to a severe pain in her shoulder that she'd been ignoring for months. Her doctor told her that anyone else enduring the kind of pain she was suffering would have been in his office months before, and said she needed surgery immediately. She mused to me that perhaps she had actually been stoic to a degree that she had disabled herself. Seeing only one side of her stoicism, ignoring her pain, had led her away from caring for herself.

What comes to mind when we think of compassion? We probably consider words like *empathy for others, caring,* or *thoughtfulness*? Wouldn't we like to feel compassionate as much as possible? Compassion is a good thing, right?

I remember a white-water-rafting trip with family members a long time ago. Our young daughter was in the raft with my husband and me and one of the guides. We all had on our life preservers, and the water was flowing, but not extremely rapidly. Still, our daughter was very fearful and could not overcome her anxiety or enjoy the experience at all. We were on the raft for the trip, and there was no way to get off. My own worries for my daughter led me to continually try to reassure her. I felt compassion for her predicament. However, my own actions seemed to further lock her into her fear. Looking back, I realize that just allowing her to find her own way to deal with her fear might have been a better course of action for both of us. Sometimes when people are trying to pull themselves together, they may need space more than they need sympathy. Being compassionate may actually add to their discomfort, rather than comfort them.

And what about helpfulness? Ask a social worker if they like being helpful. That's part of what our profession is all about. Being helpful can be extremely gratifying. Working with older people offers me lots of opportunities to be helpful. The "other side" of helpfulness can be interpreted as not helping, or it could be judged as allowing another person to function as independently as possible. I regularly grapple with this issue. When is it appropriate to offer assistance, and when should I step back and let clients fend for themselves? Sometimes I make the right choice, and sometimes I don't. If a client is propelling herself in her wheelchair down a long hallway, I might ask if she wants a push or would rather do it herself. When I've offered to buy groceries for a mostly independent woman, have I overstepped and taken away her chance to do this task herself?

Helping definitely has two sides to it. Because I know I gain a lot of pleasure from helping, it warrants a good, hard look at what it may be like for the "help-ee." I often consciously accept help from clients in an effort to attempt to achieve some balance in our relationship.

It has occurred to me that we could practice this yin and yang thinking anytime. We could take minutes out of a day to examine our thoughts and actions over that time. We could consider an internal dialogue, asking ourselves, *What is the other side of those thoughts and actions?* Ten minutes of time would probably be plenty of time to try going back and forth.

Practicing this ancient Chinese way of looking at our lives, we may find that our sense of perception may have no boundaries. People I speak with about aging express fear about the limitations that aging may bring. As we get older, we will experience limitations. Discovering this yin and yang point of view can allow us to remove limits on how we think about things. Trying to envision both sides, to see the yin and yang, offers us a useful way to broaden our thinking no matter our age.

Acknowledgements

It is impossible to name all the people in my life who have encouraged and supported me in the process of writing this book. Friends, family and my dear children have listened, advised and sustained me all along the way. Thank you for all those breakfasts, phone calls, e-mails and receptive ears.

There are some professionals without whom I could never have stayed the course. Linda Cashdan was crucial at the beginning. She told me she thought I had a book. Then Gerry Sindell taught me to think like a writer and got me believing I actually *was* a writer. Thanks to Leanne Sindell for all her advice about the publishing world. I'm not sure how to account for my luck in having Bob Asher look at my manuscript, do a complete edit (!) and affirm my project. His timing was impeccable.

As much as I've grown to love words, I find I cannot find the right ones to thank my husband, Jim, for his extraordinary contribution to this book. He's been my reader, proofer, lawyer, ballast: my everything.